The International Library of Psychology

ART AND THE UNCONSCIOUS

Founded by C. K. Ogden

The International Library of Psychology

GENERAL PSYCHOLOGY
In 38 Volumes

ART AND THE UNCONSCIOUS

A Psychological Approach to a Problem of Philosophy

JOHN M THORBURN

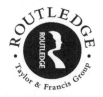

First published in 1925 by
Kegan Paul, Trench, Trubner & Co., Ltd.

Reprinted in 1999, 2001 by
Routledge
2 Park Square, Milton Park, Abingdon, Oxfordshire OX14 4RN
711 Third Avenue, New York, NY 10017

First issued in paperback 2014

*Routledge is an imprint of the Taylor and Francis Group,
an informa company*

Transferred to Digital Printing 2006

© 1925 John M Thorburn

The publishers have made every effort to contact authors/copyright holders
of the works reprinted in the *International Library of Psychology*.
This has not been possible in every case, however, and we would
welcome correspondence from those individuals/companies
we have been unable to trace.

These reprints are taken from original copies of each book. In many cases
the condition of these originals is not perfect. The publisher has gone to
great lengths to ensure the quality of these reprints, but wishes to point
out that certain characteristics of the original copies will, of necessity, be
apparent in reprints thereof.

British Library Cataloguing in Publication Data
A CIP catalogue record for this book
is available from the British Library

Art and the Unconscious
ISBN 978-0-415-21043-0 (hbk)
ISBN 978-0-415-75808-6 (pbk)

General Psychology: 38 Volumes
ISBN 978-0-415-21129-1
The International Library of Psychology: 204 Volumes
ISBN 978-0-415-19132-6

ANALYTICAL TABLE OF CONTENTS

PART I

CHAPTER I

The Selective Meditation of the Artist

TABLE OF CONTENTS

TABLE OF CONTENTS

Chapter III

Plasticity and Vision

TABLE OF CONTENTS

CHAPTER IV

Vision and Convention

CHAPTER V

The Transition to Music

viii

TABLE OF CONTENTS

CHAPTER VI

Art as the Relation of Outer and Inner

TABLE OF CONTENTS

TABLE OF CONTENTS

TABLE OF CONTENTS

PART I

THE PSYCHOLOGY OF THE
ARTISTIC PROCESS

Art as the formulation of an unique and distinct psychological
attitude is unquestionably ONE.

EDWARD BULLOUGH.

ART AND THE UNCONSCIOUS

CHAPTER I

THE SELECTIVE MEDITATION OF THE ARTIST

Art . . . is an expression of the reflective and fully conscious life.
ROGER FRY

> Oh ! Mensch ! Gieb Acht !
> Was spricht die tiefe Mitternacht ?
> " Ich schlief, ich schlief—
> Aus tiefem Traum bin ich erwacht :—
> Die Welt ist tief
> Und tiefer als der Tag gedacht."
> NIETZSCHE

I PROPOSE in the following pages to ask how far the problem of art and the sources of its inspiration may be re-stated in the light of those discoveries of contemporary Psychology which centre round what has been called, significantly enough, the Unconscious. Of the significance of the name I entertain no doubt, nor need any honest inquirer of whatever mode of thinking. Yet significance is not necessarily the equivalent of accuracy ; and the accuracy of the term in its general application has received the most rigorous challenge alike from the side of the scientists and from the side of the artists. Questions of accurate and legitimate usage thus immediately arise and force us to state the problem in terms that lead back to the central problems of æsthetic, and, indeed, of philosophy itself.

The relevant conceptions of Schopenhauer, of Bosanquet, of Ruskin, form an integral part of the present discussion ; and it would be undesirable, with

3

due regard to the relative importance of issues, not to make special mention of the precision of the lead given by Mr. Edward Bullough to the Science of Æsthetic. Nevertheless, it must be made clear at the outset, these thinkers are invoked only in so far as the conceptions they have elaborated appear to furnish us with a means of approach to the new problem, or to the problem as set in its new terms. One must, I think, go a little further than that and even estimate the conceptions of these thinkers by the extent to which the new psychological discoveries prove their validity and give them illumination.

Speculation as to the nature of art has traditionally been evaded by philosophy, sometimes being regarded as more difficult, sometimes as less significant than other problems of philosophy. It has received less than its due attention, on the whole perhaps because of its inherent remoteness from anything that could be called science. Art cannot, of course, become accessible to the scientist without first convincing him of its beauty. The work of art that is not felt to be beautiful cannot, as art, become a datum of science. Yet the beauty of art may very well be accessible to the scientist in a new way; or his experience of its beauty may be held in review by him through a new method. Certainly the significance of art for science has *changed*; and if it has changed for science, it has changed, too, for philosophy. If art has become less remote from science, it has become less remote from philosophy.

The discoveries of Freud and subsequent investigators are among the most wonderful and fascinating that the history of European culture can show. Perhaps, also, they give a profounder view of nature than anything that has been given hitherto, at all events, by science. Be that as it may, it is through these discoveries that science now begins to have

4

a real approach to art. The inscrutable shapes and divine phantasms of art are recognised at last by their kinship with ' The Unconscious.'

Art, however, is a sphere of life to which common humanity has access with an immediacy, with a freedom and with a delight that the new psychological movement has not yet fully taken into account. That movement has made its approach to art, knowing itself to be in possession of a wonderful secret ; in this knowledge, it would explore the field of art in quest of more and more material for its own enlightenment and for its own purposes, extraneous to those of art. In some respects it may have gained these ends, but in others there is a danger that the very wealth and resources of its own knowledge and ıe security of its own standpoint should make it blind to some essential qualities of the experience it proposes to scrutinise. We need the new psychological method in its application to an artist's work, not primarily to explain the aberrations of his temperament ; but because it is worth while more deeply to understand the nature of art itself, and to see its value in true perspective with the other values of life. If our reading of art in terms of ' the unconscious ' is to have significance, it cannot be by regarding art only as a phenomenon that a new psychological method can analyse and explain— perhaps, explain away—as a mere by-product. The application to art of a psychology of the unconscious can have significance only in relation to a problem of value—of value in art itself, first of all, but in relation as well, to other values. The true significance of the concept of the unconscious lies, then, in regarding it as a key to the problem of value.

Once again the mention of the term unconscious gives us pause. For, on the one hand, it means something real. It cannot, through the misunderstanding of a vain and arid criticism, merely be discarded. On the other hand, there is no little justification for the observation that " the looseness with which the word ' unconscious ' is at present used is a psychological scandal of the first magnitude."[1] That, then, would be our first difficulty—to leave room for the reality of the fact, whatever it be, implied by the term, while exercising some sort of safeguard against hypnotism by a word.

I do not, therefore, propose to start by assuming an ' unconscious,' though I have to reiterate my conviction that the term means something worth meaning. I should attempt, rather, to state an initial point of view based on the incontrovertible proposition that people do indeed have dreams, in an absolutely simple and unmetaphorical sense of the word. That is the basal psychological fact.

Some poems have indisputable likeness to dreams —the *Divina Comedia*, to give an obvious example, and perhaps, too, some of the minor poems of Dante. The name which Carey gave to his translation of the *Comedia*, " The Vision of Dante," has always presented itself to me as more than a felicitous title ; and I think we may take Ruskin as expressing the *consensus gentium* in the matter when he says of the *Comedia*, " It is indeed a vision, but a vision only and that one of the wildest that ever entranced a human soul . . ." Dante, we may conceive, could easily pass from dream to poem. There is so undeniably present the wildness and the strangeness and the chaos of the dream in much of his writing ; and the beautiful sonnet in the *Vita Nuova* about " the lord of great and terrible aspect " is itself supposed to be the telling of a dream. It is not difficult to imagine that Dante could incorporate

[1] *Various Meanings of the Term Unconscious.* C. D. Broad. Aristotelian Society Proceedings, April 9th, 1923.

his dreams in his poetry without always being clear which were the dream and which the poem.

Not all poetry gives us such a marked resemblance to dreams as that of Dante ; nor are those poets whose work bears the most dream-like character always willing, as readily as Dante, to admit this aspect of their art. Thus Mallarmé whose short lyrics are a sort of exquisite mystery with sometimes as little intelligible meaning as the strangest of dreams speaks of the dream as inimical to the task devolving upon the poet of guarding the paradise of his art.[1]

Granting, however, that dreams may obtrude themselves in a poet's work in such fashion as to mar it, it does not follow—it is even contradicted by the character of Mallarmé's own work—that the poem bears no relation to the dream. It might be quite true that poetry is " such stuff as dreams are made of," and yet some poems might be so made with skill or genius, others with feebleness—ineffectually wrought, yet of the same material.

Again, extending the scope of our inquiry to art, we might find some pictures or some music extraordinarily dream-like in character, others far less so, others perhaps having at least no superficial or obvious resemblance to dreams. If, however, as the presupposition of our whole argument runs, " art as the formulation of an unique and distinct psychological attitude is unquestionably one," must it not follow that, if some art conveys an irresistible impression of being like a dream, all art may in the last resort demand interpretation through the same analogy ?

We shall proceed, then, to inquire if the analogy between art and dream will hold good in every sphere,

[1] . . . le poète pur a pour geste humble et large
De l'interdire au rêve, ennemi de sa charge.

and for every kind of art ; and if so, how far it will explain or interpret experience of beauty. It should be remembered, however, that this analogy would constitute our initial, not our final view of the problem. The experience of dreams is one that seems more or less, if not entirely, to rule out conscious direction and control. Dreams come unwilled and are natural phenomena rather than products of individuality. Genius, however spontaneous, however apparently effortless, is always individual ; and art, if it be worth the name, is usually taken to be one of the highest expressions of individuality. The analogy, therefore, however significant we may find it, is bound to leave us with some of the essentials of art unaccounted for, in the last resort. We may not, for that reason, refuse to avail ourselves of the power of the analogy.

The initial presentation of such an analogy as that between art and dream must, in the very nature of the case, be indistinct and blurred in outline. It is necessary to pay this price, so that the things that are massive and that really are in possession of the momentum that counts may loom in due relative proportion within the view. We can only attempt to bring it gradually into focus, allowing definition and articulation to come slowly. Such a focussing of the initial view can do no more than leave the way open for succeeding chapters where greater clearness and more precise formulation may become possible.

(I)

The dream is first of all an expression of something that cannot find its way into our waking life, or, at least, that cannot find admittance there with any degree of clearness or energy. At the same time, it is obvious that the material of our dreams is partly drawn from the events and activities of the day before, or even of the weeks or months before.

How, then, is the dream related to the preceding experience in waking life ? Analytical study of the dream has shown that it goes away back to the infantile, and perhaps to the pre-natal past. This is the profound discovery around which, after all, our discussion must turn. But it is not only legitimate, it is also an obvious necessity of our method, to ask in the first place about the relation of dreams to the more immediately preceding conscious experience. It is a matter that is difficult to formulate. I should point first to the essential community of content between the dream and the waking life that goes before it. I admit that I stumble over the word, ' content.' It is, of course, easy to show that an object noticed during the day may re-appear in the dream by night, and so far there is undoubted community of content. To speak, however, of intellectual concepts as content or material that enters afresh into the dream is more dangerous ; but we must certainly have some means of saying that ideas entertained during the day do in some way influence or limit the dream by night. With the reservations thus indicated, then, I think we are bound to assert that our waking hours and our dreams have such a common content.

For a dream is the counterpart of an attitude. When a man is called upon to choose from a number of possible modes of action, his choice of one course involves the exclusion of the others. With a few rare exceptions, men cannot in general have two professions. If a lad chooses to be a sailor, he cannot at the same time be a musician. The decision, with its intention to make good along the chosen pathway, rules out many faculties of mind—those in especial that make it at least worth while to think of making music his life-work. Decision thus involves repression; or repression is the negative side of decision. Perhaps not every decision involves repression of an obvious kind. Yet some decisions do. There is a certain kind of intention that does not admit of the use of even cherished gifts. In so far, at all events, as decision and intention involve repression, there we find the dream, or the tendency to dream. In this sense, then, the dream is the counterpart of an attitude.

The strength of decision and the persistence of intention which condition an attitude, are integrally bound up with ideas. A thing is judged to be good on the ground, it may be, of a very elaborate ideal construction. Ideal construction, at all events, is *one* of the things that as often as not go hand in hand with attitude. It does not matter at all for our purpose in the meantime whether idea conditions attitude or *vice versa*, or whether each reinforces the other. All we need to show is the concomitance of the two. On the one hand, then, we have the attitude of consciousness towards life, or a certain side of life, with its counter-part in the so-called unconsciousness of the dream.

Let us try to work this out in a more concrete fashion.

Suppose a man is inwardly dissatisfied with the ethical and religious conceptions current in his time, or upon which he has been content hitherto to base his life. Suppose that on reflection he arrives at new ideas, more or less definite, and that he brings these into distinct relation to his activities. The character of the latter is altered, and that consciously. The change of conduct is the result of deliberate resolution. As we saw, any such resolution involves choice and will necessitate the renunciation of several otherwise desirable or profitable activities or modes of action. Now, though the man may have been right to discard the old orientation to life, there may remain minor aspects of the discarded attitude that had value and whose value it is a mistake to ignore. Yet in the elation of a new discovery, he does ignore them. It is a world-old situation. It is something that may happen—perhaps ought to happen—to every son of human race.

The eagerness, we had supposed, with which he launches himself upon the new plan makes him oblivious of many things in the old and discarded scheme of things that it had been really worth his while to remember. Of the loss of the things thus too inconsiderately jettisoned, he may have some elusive sensibility or half-consciousness. It causes him, perhaps, some vague and indefinite disquietude of spirit.

But the new plan itself need not be vague ; it may be clearly conscious, as clearly conscious as anything can be. The new intention may be credited with all the attributes of consciousness, and that without any sort of ambiguity. It is the result of intellectual reflection, and it is carried into effect by acts of will. At length, however, there comes the time of day, or of evening, or of night, when the working out of the plan has to be relinquished. Sleep comes, and in sleep the dream.

Sleep comes. We say, one *falls* asleep. There is, then, first, a falling—a movement downwards. And it *is* a falling, a helpless, delightful loss of control over every kind of action ; and the deeper one falls, the more passive does one become.

One falls asleep, and dreams. One lapses or glides down into a strange form of experience—strange because of its remoteness from what we lightly and familiarly term experience.

ART AND THE UNCONSCIOUS

In the dream there is certainly something very passive. There is a quiet—as it were, evasive and unobserved—renunciation of that difficult mode of experience which proceeds by concepts, and a pleased acceptance of that easier mode which proceeds through images. There is passivity, and extreme passivity ; and yet that is not quite all.

It is, I confess, a matter of never-ceasing wonder to me that we can go to sleep—and dream. Other marvels of the universe become stale by repetition, but surely never the dream. What I most admire in it is the ceaseless activity of the people and the monsters that one meets there, and sometimes, too, the ingenuity and originality in oneself, the dreamer. The people and the monsters of the dream—its denizens, as we say—are not passive. Very active, they. It is not enough, therefore, to think of the dream only as a gliding and a falling downward into passivity. We must also admit that here something that has not had its innings in the daylight springs up into activity in the night. We might say that a capacity for life that we have ignored takes its revenge and secures its experience in spite of us. Where the activity comes in, however, is rather in what I have called the denizens of the dream. Each is its own little centre of activity ; and they often fight with each other ; and they seem to be fighting *about* something as often as not. It is as if each were out to get his own share of life and experience and to dispute anyone or anything that challenged his right.

For our purpose, then, the dream seems to have two main characteristics. First of all, the denizens of the dream are ' real ' people or monsters. By real, I mean that they are not inventions, or in any sense artificial. They manifest that unique power of initiation that belongs alone to living things.

They are centres of vitality whose self-motion is not to be controlled by the dreamer. They act at variance with his wishes ; and when, by some rare chance, the lady of his dreams is gracious, she is so entirely of her own accord and through her own individuality, and not remotely in virtue of anything he may desire. That is to say, the denizens of the dream are at the extreme opposite of anything like a logical fabrication. The best of novelists or playwrights occasionally lapses into a logical fabrication, or is guilty of a logically consistent heroine. The dream, never. All in that realm are themselves, exactly as the Almighty created them, and they show no trace of the artificially devising touch of man.

In the second place, the dream is a unity—a dramatic unity—a real unity of action. At first sight and in view of the apparently chaotic and bewildering confusion of the dream to the rational consciousness of the awakened dreamer, this may seem paradoxical. But let us go for a moment to dramatic art to help us, through its analogy, in the elucidation of this aspect of the dream. In the first impression made by many finely constructed plays, the inner unity of the successive presentations of the action need not easily emerge. At first, the contrast presented by successive scenes may seem like that between two entirely different episodes of history having no connection with each other. The essential relation emerges only when the impression is deepened at the cost, perhaps, of very great concentration on the part of the spectator. It is even the skill of the playwright not too easily or cheaply to exhibit the relation of the scenes. In the dream, the inner relation between the parts of its action is of the same kind, but apprehended with greater difficulty by the dreamer when he awakes to the scrutiny of his dream. The dream often falls apart into scenes, or presentations of its *motif*, that appear to have no connection with each other. Only upon considerable effort, upon concentration on the impression of the dream, and careful search for the associations of its several parts, does their integral relation to each other begin to emerge. And, of course, just as there are badly constructed plays that contain irrelevant and non-dramatic material, there are, conceivably vague, and uncertain dreams presenting more doubtfully this characteristic unity. Such dreams are perhaps the correlates of a vacillating and uncertain conscious attitude.

A certain degree of unity in the dream is, then, required before the vitality and the individuality of its denizens can be brought out in their interplay with each other and with the dreamer. Individual though they be, they are so only in and through the story of the dream, or rather the action of the dream ; for the dream is, on the whole, nearer the dramatic than the historical or narrative. And in passing it might be remarked that the closer approximation of dramatic art to the dream has an important bearing on literary theory. If, as it has often been maintained, the drama is essentially superior to the novel as a form of art, it may not be altogether beside the mark to attempt to explain its superiority through its closer resemblance to the dream.

Let us go back now to the picture we were attempting to sketch of a man trying to find a new approach to life and a better reading of experience through his religious and ethical concepts. We thought of him as excited by the novelty of his discovery, and we could easily conceive that such eagerness in the *vita nuova* would create a kind of tension within him all day long ; as though he had kept himself in a state of spiritual or psychical strain and had become like a bow that is only held bent by continuous expenditure of energy and but awaits the opportunity when the energy shall be withdrawn, by a vigorous reaction to become straight again. And because of that over-tension, we know, when he goes to sleep, he will dream. That much we do know. But at this point we are confronted with a difficulty of the most formidable character. For we have to ask, how far can an idea of conscious and deliberate reflection that is directed towards a practical end, and that dominates the mind perhaps for many days and weeks, pass into, and mould the form of a dream by night ? I prefer to say "mould the form of " rather than to say "pass into "; because, of course, neither the dominating idea nor any parts of it need survive in the dream as idea. And yet to say "mould the form of " is not quite enough, because that seems to imply only a kind of limitation of the dream by the idea. This is the paradox of the matter. For the ideas of conscious life vanish utterly as ideas when a man descends into the depths of sleep ; and yet it is not true to say that the ideas of waking reflection do nothing more than mould the form of our dreams. I should like to say, rather, they become the very fabric and stuff of our dreams, save that 'fabric' and 'stuff' are too metaphorical to be of any use. So I had rather rest content with the negative form—that while ideas conceived in our waking life vanish utterly as ideas, it is not enough to say that they merely influence, or mould the form of our dreams.

Again, in whatever way the ideas of waking life survive in the dream, or whatever aspect of them is preserved, it is clear that their practical value is lost. In sleep we are deprived of power to act. I think we can trace the real meaning of this aspect of the dream through the phantasy or day-dream.

When we build castles in the air, we do not act ; we shall never act. Dreaming, then, is castle-building in the air—intensive castle building, we might call it, and doubly remote from all chances of action. There is only the activity of the denizens of the dream ; and there is the motion, the movement, the *motif* of the dream in which their activities unite and which their activities sustain and create.

I should attempt, then, to summarise this part of the argument somewhat as follows. The advent of sleep deprives the idea conceived in conscious life of all possibility of carrying itself into effect in practice. But instead of being applied to practical life, it seems somehow to give unity to the activity of the people of the dream. It is in the dying of the idea as a practical possibility that these little people live their lives and experience their individualities. Discussion of the other side of the analogy—that of art—may afterwards help us to bring into clearer focus this view of the dream in relation to consciousness. Yet we must meantime formulate a tentative conclusion, viz., That to the unity discoverable in an attitude of conscious reflection and deliberate plan, there can be found a correlate in the unity which appears in the dream and finds expression in the characters of the dream.

Let us turn now to the other side of the analogy—that of art and literature.

(2)

The art of literature, or even that part of it which can, without reserve, be placed within the sphere of the fine arts in the strictest sense, presents unique difficulties to the student of æsthetic, and at the same time, in virtue of these very difficulties, is peculiarly rich in suggestion towards a theory of beauty. For literature, or even poetry, in the narrowest sense, bears the form of language. Language is the instrument of the intellect and it is in the typical employment of language that we think we are most entirely conscious. Language, we might say, is the form of the conscious.

And yet in poetry, we feel, language tends to abrogate its intellectual and practical powers. If the intellect be present, it is present rather as falling within a larger and non-intellectual whole. It is present, sometimes, in subordination to an intention that not merely ignores, but even runs athwart, all real intellectual values. It will be said against this that Lucretius in the writing of *De Rerum Natura* had a real intellectual intention. What confronts us, however, is not so much the kinship of Lucretius to the philosopher as his kinship to the author of a *Midsummer Night's Dream*, who declared that " the best in this kind are but shadows and the worst are no worse an imagination amend them." Sometimes, in poetry, we are bound to say, the intellect is subservient to a non-intellectual intention ; and if this subservience be a real quality of poetry anywhere must it not be so everywhere ?

We cannot at present define this intention ; but we might legitimately suppose that it is an intention well exhibited also in the other arts and perhaps especially in music. Music, or at all events that kind of music which has moved away from all dependence on the human voice, seems peculiarly free from the bondage of the intellect, and therefore there is a natural inclination to suppose that music exhibits the non-intellectual, perhaps the non-conscious, intention of art better than poetry. In some respects it may do this ; in other respects perhaps not ; and so far we are justified in supposing that poetry, notwithstanding its *soi-disant* intellectual form, is able to free itself from the bondage of the intellect in as real a sense as any of the other arts. If, therefore, art is something that in Nietzsche's language, takes us down into the depths of the world, we may have access to those depths as well in poetry as in any other kind of art.

In view of the *soi-disant* intellectual form of poetry, it is natural that theories should have arisen which vested the poetical worth of literature in its truth. It may be that, in point of psychological fact, intellect and literary power are found united more frequently than intellect and other forms of artistic power. I should think that this is so, though it is perhaps a disputable view. What is not in the least open to dispute is the difference between the social environment from which arises the greatest music and the environment that begets poetry and the drama in their most typical magnificence. The education and training to which the poet falls heir, under the cultural conditions of Europe, differ almost *toto coelo* from those bestowed upon the generality of other artists. It cannot, for example, be questioned, that in England, literary and musical tradition have fallen strangely—I had said disastrously—apart, were it not that the implication of disaster unduly complicates the argument. At all events, whether for well or ill, music in England has been altogether beyond the scope and vision of philosophy. Literature has not fallen so entirely below its horizon. In Scotland, much the same is true. Music, for the purposes of our argument, may be regarded as non-existent ; while Scottish intellectual tradition keeps, as it were, a kind of shrewd touch with the literary. In point of psychological fact, then, poetry falls together with the intellect, to an extent not at all shared by the other arts. With the still doubtful exception of Germany, musical and literary tradition fall very far apart. Even Goethe, whom in point of universality of artistic and cultural interests, " few sons of men may think to emulate," once said that music was not his province.

Now that tradition of æsthetic theory which has had by far the greatest influence in our island, viz., the Hegelian, has originated in a soil and thrives in a climate where the cultural convergence of literature and philosophy has been most marked. It is very natural, then, that an Æsthetic thus traditionally grounded should still continue to look for the value of poetry as though it were to be found in its truth, and then to extend the conception to other forms of art.

It is simple enough for facile expressionist theories to point out the obvious error in such a view. It is perhaps not so simple for them to preserve the rich and fruitful suggestion of the older theories.

Language is the form of consciousness ; and though poetry conserves this form only in appearance, not in reality, this apparent preservation of the intellectual form is one of the things that distinguishes poetry from the other arts. It is just this apparent continuation of the intellectual in a non-intellectual form of experience that gives æsthetic inquiry a cue far too important and valuable to ignore. It is of this fact that we must find means to discover the real bearing.

Emphasis is, indeed, placed upon it both by popular feeling towards poetry and by critical usage. We are not too wide of the mark when we praise poetry for its depth of thought. Are not Æschylus, Dante, Goethe and Keats significantly characterised by their depth of thought ? Yet this significance, real as it is, may require a re-interpretation. For the apparent thought-content of poetry—an appearance so much more striking than in the case of the other arts—led the older idealistic theorists to speak as if they could start from it, and develop it and relate it to other intellectual matters ; to speak as if they could isolate it and oppose it to some other perhaps non-intellectual element in poetry ; and yet to speak as if all the æsthetic worth of poetry lay in the value of the idea which they thus thought to isolate. The expressionist or allied theories are clearly right in so far as they protest against this supposed isolation of an idea. And yet my feeling always has been that the expressionists miss the deepest and the most interesting and the most real thing about poetry and the arts. They are unable to relate the arts to life. They are unable to say how the arts came to be, or to trace the psychological path along which the artist passes from his own experience of men and women and nature to his creative work as artist. Not knowing how art arises out of life, they are unable to say what effect it has upon life, and how great works of art influence the subsequent generations whose heritage they are. But the things that happen in a man's experience, before he reaches a purely artistic accomplishment on the one hand, and the way in which the accomplishment affects other men and leads them beyond and outside anything that can properly be called art on the other— these are things of supreme importance. They are also of very great interest. But the supremacy of their importance, over and above their interest, lies in the fact that they condition the approach of the artist to his art. Now it is the conditioning of that approach—the attitude—which gives vitality to the art. When it is said that a poet sings not because he will, but because he must, it is usually said in praise ; and it is taken for granted that the singing is so far forth the better because he cannot help it. This is the statement of a vital attitude. How are we to describe and interpret that attitude and the vitality of the poetry it begets ?

Or again, it is a commonplace that a poet cannot write before he has lived. True, there is the antithesis between ' the poetry of phantasy ' and ' the poetry of experience ; ' but even the poetry of phantasy requires a certain background of life ; while in the case of the greater dramatic poets, the impression created by their tragic power leads us irresistibly away from their art back to the story of their life. And where history cannot furnish us with much material, where the personality of the author has become shadowed in oblivion " like the tradition of a lost heathen god," we try to reconstruct his personality from whatever sources we may. This is how we testify to our conviction of the importance of the poet's experience of life, *vis-à-vis* his art.

Or, finally, it has been the experience of many a poet that until he has thought, he cannot come to his own in poetry. As a rule, there is but little chance of confusion between the thought-experience and the poetic experience. The letters of Keats show traces of profound thinking, but they are entirely different from his poetic work. We need the former to understand the latter, that is all.

Summarising these illustrations in general terms : poetry is a highly differentiated form of experience that in virtue of its very differentiation cannot be confused with non-æsthetic forms of experience, in themselves often clearly differentiated along quite other lines. But while so easily distinguishable, the æsthetic and the non-æsthetic are closely related ; and the formulation of the inter-dependence and inter-relation may often be a task of extreme complexity. It is only through such a formulation that we can discover the attitude of the poet to his art—the criterion of what is vital in his work.

The same is true of the other arts. It is more difficult, however, to formulate their relation to the experience out of which they arise, than in the case of literature. There may be many practical reasons

connected with the tradition and technique of literature why its riddle should be a little easier to read.
But, by a stricter logic, the apparently intellectual
form that belongs to poetry is the specific cue that
must be followed, first in contrasting it with the other
arts, and then in applying to them what can be discerned from the scrutiny of poetry. Poetry thus
appears to set a special line of investigation that
cannot be evaded. Afterwards, any real æsthetic
facts apprehended in this sphere should be applicable
to the other spheres of art and should reveal in them
the correlated facts far more easily than is possible
by a more immediate investigation.

It is, therefore, with the art of poetry specially in
mind that we make our initial statement of the
problem of art. The topic of this chapter—the
scrutiny of the pathway by which the literary artist
arrives at the creative period of his work—will, it is
suggested, afford a key to the more difficult form that
the investigation is bound to assume in the sphere of
the other arts. In theoretical principle, there is, in
this respect, no difference between any of the arts ;
in point of æsthetic method and convenience of
approach to the problem each in turn may present,
the difference is marked.

Meanwhile a contrast is drawn, or an antithesis is
indicated, between a phase of selective meditation
and a moment of creative *élan*.

(3)

Let us, then, try to hold in relation the life and
experience of some of the greater poets to their art,
noting the general features of the pathway along
which they went before they actually wrote the poem
or the play. Shakespeare and Goethe invite our

attention in a very special way ; for these two poets of the modern world, whether by natural temperament or by favour of outer circumstances, were placed in a position of extraordinary advantage to form rich and abundant relationships with men and women of all ranks and of all types of natural endowment. Both poets lived much about courts and had much of the courtier in them. Shakespeare was an actor by profession, and a man of much practical efficiency in the conduct of affairs. So was Goethe. If not an actor, he, too, had much practical contact with the stage, and he had something very like Shakespeare's efficiency in the handling of the least artistic elements of life.

A pretty clear distinction, however, is visible between the two men, inasmuch as Goethe was a scientist and philosopher, which Shakespeare was not. Again, we know that before any important course of action, Goethe reflected a very long time. The distance between Shakespeare's reflection and his action was probably a very much shorter one. Still more relevant to our purpose is the fact that Goethe reflected a great deal about the nature of art ; Shakespeare did not.

From this last consideration, it is clear that Goethe's critical and reflective writing would be of the most immediate service to our problem. On the other hand, the sharper antithesis between Shakespeare's contemplative vision in poetry and Shakespeare, the man of action, states the problem in more simple terms. What Goethe has done for himself in the general autobiographical character of so much of his writing, it requires some other and external observer to do for Shakespeare. Professor A. C. Bradley, for example, in *Shakespearian Tragedy* has done this for the English poet, and he has done it supremely well.

I am the more content, in my approach to the

subject of tragedy and tragic poetry, to follow Bradley, because of his insistence on the conditioning of tragic impression through moral factors. It still seems to me true to say that always the consciousness of a moral order is to be found somewhere in the poet, implied by his work. In spite of all that has been said against moralistic theories of art, I cannot get beyond this, that all tragedy and all great tragic poetry exhibit somewhere the recognition of a moral order. It may be, of course, that it is through the poet's sense of his own violation of this order that we get the best results, as in the case of the more dissolute of the Elizabethan dramatists, or *par excellence* in François Villon. But that scarcely affects the main contention.

There is a remarkable passage in Ruskin indicating the mode in which the perfectness of the tragic spirit is conditioned by the poet's recognition of the moral order. He compares Dante and Milton, on the one hand, who seem just to fall short of the tragic spirit, with Homer and Shakespeare on the other, who achieve it absolutely and in its entirety. He conceives the first two as " unable to discern where their own ambition modified their utterance of the moral law ; or their agony mingled with anger at its violation." Of the two latter, Homer and Shakespeare, he speaks as of men " to whose unoffended, uncondemning sight, the whole of human nature reveals itself in a pathetic weakness, with which they will not strive ; or in mournful and transitory strength which they dare not praise." And so he adds, significantly, " all pagan and Christian civilisation thus become subject to them." That theme—the subjection of civilisation to the tragic poet—is the counterpart of our present topic, its complement, indeed, and not separable from it. The temporal

24

succession of the critical and appreciative attitude to the creative act may, however, justify the logic of putting it aside in the meantime.

In illustrating through such types as Shakespeare and Goethe, it is natural that the ethical side of the matter should leap into prominence. For the personal and spiritual history of both poets is one which has never ceased to command the interest of their readers from their own day to ours. Need it be so for every poet ? I do not want to limit poetry. There may be an infinitude of things that condition poetry besides the recognition of what I have called, for the sake of brevity, the moral order. It is but for simplicity that I confine myself meantime to the single aspect ; but I do think that with regard to dramatic poetry, at all events, it is important. It may even be found that tragedy can be defined with a certain precision through this aspect. This narrower question need not, however, at present be raised. The issue that I am meantime concerned to state comprehends much more than tragedy strictly so-called ; and it is on the broader ground that I venture to outline my typical case. For I am trying to *typify* the relation of conscious idea to the unity of the poem.

By " conscious idea " I mean something external to the poem in the sense that it belongs to the poet, not as poet, but as man ; and is believed by him as a matter of personal conviction, or is elaborated in his mind as a matter of personal urgency. By " poem " I mean to include the novel and the prose drama. The inclusion is legitimate in so far at least as one of my illustrations is from a Russian author, in whose case this use of the word, poem, would be natural in a sense that it cannot be for the English reader.

In speaking of the dream, I tried to show that it is possible to correlate an idea conceived or elaborated in conscious and waking hours with a dream and its imagery ; and that the idea may in some way be absorbed in these. So now in approaching the topic of art, I am trying to show that it is possible to correlate an idea thus consciously conceived or an attitude thus defined in thought with a poem or a play and the characters that appear in it.

In dealing with the dream side of our analogy, our discussion, it will be remembered, fell into two parts, closely inter-related, indeed, but distinguishable for the purposes of exposition. The first part was concerned with the vitality and individuality of the denizens of the dream, the second with its unity. In dealing with the art side of our analogy, we can adopt, not indeed a precisely corresponding arrangement, but one that will serve to bring out the relation of the idea, first, to the characters of the poem, second, to its unity. These relations are, of course, inter-dependent ; or rather they are not two, but one. In illustrating the two inter-dependent parts, I shall choose for the first, the case of Dostoevsky, for the second the poem of Dante.

Meantime, however, let us try to make a concrete statement of the problem in an idiom somewhat similar to that which was employed in elaborating the relation of idea to dream.

Suppose the poet or the literary artist to have certain ideas about social development and religion. He may be a thinker, or potentially a thinker. There are times, at all events, when he may reflect about these things in a severely intellectual way. Perhaps he is also a man of practical capacity and wishes his ideas to take effect within the society where he finds himself. Or if he be not himself a politician, he believes in his own ideas as of political worth, given over into the hands of the right people. But he is also a poet ; and as a poet or a man of letters, there is something in him that tends, as it were, to take the keen edge of the practical intellect off his ideas and to subdue them into a novel or a play. Some particular idea, let us suppose, begins to take possession of him. He has perhaps some sort of belief in social well-being or some eagerness towards revolution, or it might be, his attitude is one of affirmed scepticism towards those things. Or perhaps he is a cynic. In any of these cases, his idea will be tinged with emotion. He will naturally try to find some expression of it in a novel or a play. If so, characters will begin to form themselves and pass upon the stage of his mind's eye. If he be a real poet, these will present themselves with a certain degree of spontaneity. On the other hand, if the philosophical side of him be also fairly vigorous, is it not conceivable that there may ensue a certain conflict[1] between the philosophical development of the characters ? Let the philosophical gain a partial or complete victory ; the play would be spoilt, or simply would not come out a play at all. Suppose, on the other hand, the characters to develop with a spontaneity altogether independent of the artist's will or intention ; the play might then have a better chance of success ; but there is this danger, that the characters should develop with a delightful spontaneity to a splendid individuality, but with a vitality so strong that they should become independent of the idea. If so, what would there be to give unity to the play or the novel ? Would it not become a series of phantastic scenes, very beautiful perhaps in a sense, but not showing the dramatic structure that is essential to good literary work, or at least to the highest types of literature ? The first kind of relative imperfection seems to me to be represented

---

[1] Cf. *Distance as an Æsthetic Principle.* Edward Bullough. British Journal of Psychology, Vol. V., Part 2.

by much of our own contemporary drama where the
too consciously ethical survives at the expense of
the individuality or humanity of the characters. I
cannot help thinking that Mr. Shaw is here the chief
of sinners. If only he could lay aside the arrogance
of his own all-too-conscious points of view, and let
the divine within him have a more unhindered
utterance! Of the second relative imperfecton there
is no clearer and more significant instance than
Shelley's *Prometheus Unbound.*

As against these, can there not be a case where
the idea of ethical reflection does indeed die as the
characters emerge and develop, but where it just dies
and no more—where its death does not take place, as
it were, a moment too soon, but is nevertheless a
fact accomplished in the movement of the story?

What I have especially in mind as I formulate
this question is the instance of Dostoevsky. His
reflection and his artistic work do seem pretty well to
illustrate my typical case. Whether you will call
him philosopher or not, he certainly had aspirations
towards philosophical thinking. That he read—or
tried to read—*The Critique of Pure Reason* does not,
I think, misrepresent his mentality. His conscious
reflection was something like this: Christian ethic
had had its representation, real enough, and heroic
enough, all down the Christian ages. Yet Christian
ethic seemed in the last resort a failure, futile and
incapable of holding its own against the brute impact
of the blind forces of nature and of society. Its only
result had been the submergence or annihilation of
its best representatives. It was, therefore, only fair
to state clearly and to consider impartially the
proposition that Christian ethic was *not* suitable to
the well-being of society or to its progress, if such
there be. But as against this Dostoevsky believed
he saw in Christianity something of intrinsic value,

apart from the possibility of its successful social application. This was the form which the antimony of value took in Dostoevsky's mind, and in his conscious reflection he seems to reach a fairly clear statement of it.

Here is the point at which we begin to discover the value of the appeal to literature with its apparent intellectual form. It may quite well be that a certain emotion expressed in music has its secret origin in certain religious conceptions ; yet it is exceedingly difficult to show that a series of chords or the interweaving of melodies with which no words were ever associated, can contain or express anything even remotely akin to a religious conception. Directly to convince the sceptic in such a case is admittedly impossible. It is an entirely different proposition in the case of a novel written by a man who has elsewhere committed to writing his individual reflections about life, religion and conduct. Dostoevsky makes his characters, over and over again, and amid inconceivable varieties of circumstance, talk, on an apparent intellectual plane, on those very topics with which his own intellect was individually and vitally concerned.

It does not matter what be the form assumed by these reflections. That form may be artistic or philosophic, or what you please, so long as the writer feels the urgency of his subject. But it does matter what form be assumed by the reflections of the characters in *The Possessed*, when they talk about social theory " in Varvara Petrovna's drawing-room " or elsewhere. We must be enthralled by the story, and it must not present itself to us as moral discussion or as religion or as any other kind of thing save an all-powerful enchantment and an overwhelming tragedy.

The point at issue, then, is that when we pass

from Dostoevsky the man and the intellect to Dostoevsky as creator and literary artist, we can watch the idea of his conscious reflection become dissolved and absorbed in the action of his novels. It is perhaps best illustrated by comparing Dostoevsky's own conscious reflection on the *motif* 'Christian Ethic *versus* Social Truth,' with Ivan's parable of the Grand Inquisitor in *The Brothers Karamazov*. This *motif* has its most conscious and explicit expression in one of Dostoevsky's letters, written at a much earlier date, in which he says that if he were offered the choice between Christ and the truth, he would prefer to stay with Christ and not with the truth.

In the parable, it will be remembered, Christ is eventually rejected by the Grand Inquisitor as being incompatible with the social order. Yet Ivan Karamazov, as he relates the parable, makes the Christ kiss the Grand Inquisitor as the latter sends him out into the darkness. Ivan, I suppose, chooses the truth rather than Christ.

This passage with its terrible impressiveness is sufficiently typical of the genius of Dostoevsky to serve our purpose. The dissolution or absorption of the idea into the characters of the story, and into the symbols and imagery which these characters themselves call forth in the story within the story, takes place in such a way that it can be seen, and, as it were, observed in its change. It is as if, even after its absorption into the action and by the characters which it brings to birth, it is still there in a recognisable form. It is as if the substance of its entity had remained, though as idea it had vanished. And so it is to the apparent intellectual form of literature that we are indebted for thus exhibiting to us the continued identity of that which, as idea, has nevertheless perished.

SELECTIVE MEDITATION

Before leaving Dostoevsky, I have to express a perplexity. I had asked whether there were not a middle case between a writer like Shaw in whose work the too purely conscious ἦθος scarcely seems to have been absorbed in the life of the characters of his plays, and one like Shelley in whose *Prometheus Unbound* phantasy takes possession of the field at the expense of unity of impression ; and I answered the question by the suggestion that Dostoevsky might be such an artist. I have, however, now to raise the doubt whether Dostoevsky does not really, like Shelley—though as a more elemental individuality than Shelley—allow the awful power of some of the denizens of the dreaming mind to usurp a kind of unlawful supremacy and to destroy the totality of his artistic vision.

Mr. Middleton Murry in his study of Dostoevsky, emphasises the dream-like character of the later novels. They have the dream's bewildering chaos and the dream's absence of the sense of time. What is said in this intention is said almost entirely in praise ; nor do I think that too much is asserted of the greatness of Dostoevsky, taken as an intellectual and spiritual totality ; but I am not sure if the elemental force that issues in the writing of the novels is directed to a purely artistic effect. When Mr. Murry makes the remark that some of Dostoevsky's characters are not human, I am deeply intrigued. I do not know whether it is meant that they are infra-human or supra-human, or both. But I take it that the critic has no doubt that such characters come from a profound depth of the unconscious. So powerful do these characters become in their own individuality and reality, that they threaten the stability of any point of view from which the action of the story can be seen or apprehended as a whole. Instead of the idea being just

31

absorbed in their life, it is as if they had drunk up the idea *and more*—as if the idea had now a negative sign attached to it. In other words, through the plentitude of their own individuality, they threaten the existence of the individualty that conceived them. Like the monster in the tale of Frankenstein— but more awful—they would annihilate the mind that gave them birth. But is this art ? That it is power, or that it is elemental force let loose, none can deny. Has it the values of art ? That is a question I do not presume to answer, but it is a question I feel in duty bound to raise.

As regards the portrayal of character, then, by novel or drama, the analogy of the dream appears to place emphasis on the independence of the characters, in their development, from the will and intention of the author. It does, I think, explain the difference between the French classical stage and our own Elizabethan stage. The former is a noble exposition of the magnificent ἦθος of French civilization. Yet to us, at least, it is not so satisfying, I had almost said, so *humanly* satisfying, as the latter. I take the reason to be that in the English work—in Shakespeare and Webster, at least—the characters are allowed to develop more independently of the intentions and the conscious values of the dramatist than in the French. We are sometimes reminded, however, by a certain type of critical mind that the French stage may have a beauty that the English has not. It does, I think, better exhibit the beauty of formal relation in the structure of the play as a whole. It comes nearer to giving us the emotions that the form and symmetry of things like the Greek chorus and the relations of antithesis and balance between the choric odes alone can give. Perhaps for vitality and elemental individuality of character we should go to the English stage.

SELECTIVE MEDITATION

I hesitated, above, in using the word 'humanly,' because Caliban—something quite novel and original in literary history—is not quite human. I hesitated, too, as to whether Mr. Middleton Murry were quite justified in his unqualified admiration and awe confronted by the supra—and infra—human in Dostoevsky. Certainly Caliban is, in my stock phrase, the denizen of a dream—in Shakespeare's, such stuff as dreams are made of. It is interesting, too, to compare Shakespeare's unqualified superiority, in Caliban, over Maeterlinck in such fabrications as the Great Ancestor in *The Betrothal.* The Great Ancestor is not a living animal or monster or man—or denizen !—not yet a combination of these, but just a logical elaboration. Maeterlinck never dreamed him—only thought him out. Shakespeare, therefore, and Dostoevsky would appear to be on precisely the same plane as regards their portrayal of that which is not quite human. Yet again, I have to raise my doubt. Caliban could never overpower Shakespeare and deprive him of his pure artistic vision. I am not perfectly convinced that the same is true with regard to the awful powers in the abyss of Dostoevsky's imagination. Or yet again, I might grant to the latter that the abysses of his soul are deeper than Shakespeare's, and so, in one respect he may be greater than Shakespeare ; but I am not certain that he is so as an artist.

I think, sometimes at least, we can be certain of a superb unity of vision in Shakespeare—the security of a point of view from which the perspective is absolutely complete. When we turn, therefore, from the question of individuality of character in poetry to that of the unity of a poem, it might be natural to go to Shakespeare. As regards this topic, however, there is, I confess, for me a tremendous appeal in Dante ; not because I think him the greater poet, but because I cannot help feeling as if, without being greater, he were yet the more typical poet. It is not the superb unity of his poem only that impresses, though it is the longest poem in the world, in wh ch centrality of standpoint and harmony of vision are adequate to magnitude. Beyond that artistic unity —and as it seems to me, in the most real correlation— there is forced upon our recognition the unity of Dante's entire intellectual, ethical and religious orientation. No doubt it was a changing orientation ; and very important within it is the poet's experience of evil. I do not mean merely consciousness of sin, but a more positive and deliberative attitude towards evil or to what presented itself as evil. The same kind of attitude does, I think, emerge in Shakespeare's " expense of spirit in a waste of shame " ; and it was in some profound way, of supreme importance for his greatness as a poet. Of the whole unity of Dante's consciousness, however, there is one aspect that cannot escape the most careless observer. It is the attempt of the Christian in him to assimilate pagan thought and pagan culture in all its many-sidedness. We can trace easily enough the conflict in his reflective thinking, that this effort produced ; and with this conflict we can correlate some of the most touching and beautiful passages in the poem. There is, for example, the episode in the nineteenth and twentieth Cantos of the Paradise where the *motif* of Dante's wonder and sorrow about the souls of the great, heroic heathen who never knew of Christ, is clothed in such rapturous imagery and such poignant emotion. To this topic we must return at a later stage of our argument. Meantime, it is with another, though not unrelated, aspect of Dante's work to which I wish to call attention. It is to the unity of idea or *motif* as secured through unity of characterisation. For the figure of

34

Beatrice appears throughout the poem in a way in which no other figure or form of woman appears in any other poet's work. All the many-sidedness of the universe—of the universe in its mysterious depths and heights—is revealed through Beatrice. The Beatrice of the poem is, of course, not the real Beatrice. We need know nothing of the controversy as to whether there was or was not a real Beatrice Portinari. For our purpose it is important to emphasise that the Beatrice of the *Comedia* is essentially a personality that belongs to Dante's own soul, though doubtless having her origin in some real Beatrice. She is part of Dante—the part that reveals him to himself. To other poets belong many such woman mediators. The greater dramatists may have as many, say, roughly, as they have plays ; some of the lyric poets even as many as they have lyrics. Goethe had many minor figures of this kind. But he had two who surpassed the others in eminence —Margaret and Helena. Beatrice has no sort of rival or shadow. She is alone.

Now, I do not say that the poets in general do not show a far wider range of experience, a far greater many-sidedness in their experience, but I do see something significant in this uniqueness of Beatrice. It is she alone, I said, who reveals the secret depth of Dante's heart to himself. I ask, then, is there not a certain simplicity in the problem as set us by Dante, is there not a certain largeness of the writing which enables us to read something that the other poets have given only in miniscule ?

The essential of our general conclusion is that for a poem to be great there must be a correlated greatness in the poet's reflection about life or in his attitude towards the problems of life. Before we ever reach literary work of outstanding merit, we should expect to find some very long and carefully premeditated purpose—premeditated, perhaps, for half a life-time, or as in Dante's case, for more than that. Even in the case of Goethe, who had so many diverse artistic ambitions, and whose poetry seems to show so many diverging or even incompatible tendencies, there is to be found this unity of dominating purpose. The selective meditation which gave *Faust* as a whole, extended literally over a period of sixty years. According to Goethe's own account, the germ of the idea came to him in his twenty-first year. He finished the second part only a few months before his death. In this case, selective meditation seems to be a peculiarly apt term. It emphasises deliberate choice, the rejection of some things, the appropriation of others. Here, too, of course, selective meditation gives place to periods of creative work. No doubt the artistic imperfections of *Faust* are traceable, some of them, to this alternation of the creative and selective periods. In separate passages *Faust* reaches the deepest depths of unconsciousness ; but scarcely as a whole—not, at all events, the second part.

The principle is that if one awakes right up from a dream one can never fall back again into the same dream quite perfectly. That, no doubt, was a defect in Goethe's nature as a poet. He was not always willing to yield himself to the sleep from which alone could come the creative dreaming. He always wanted to keep one eye open to observe the creative process. We might be inclined to stigmatise this, for the poet, as the deadliest of sins, the sin of Ananias and Sapphira that wants to keep back the essential part of the price ; were it not that we have felt tempted, on the other hand, to accuse Dostoevsky of allowing the creatures of his dreaming imagination to usurp the authority of the pure artist. Can we judge between Dostoevsky and Goethe in this respect, both of whom have dreamed each in his own way the deepest dreams perhaps ever dreamed by poet ? Can we, in a word, find the *differentia* between art and dream by saying that in art the artist must somehow preserve for himself a conscious standpoint which the dreamer cannot do ? The very formulation of the question at this stage is difficult and dangerous. In the meantime we shall find a far simpler way of distinguishing between the two forms of experience by saying that dreaming is that kind of art which has no medium ; or, if it be preferred, that art is that kind of dream which expresses itself in some material medium.

For how is it that the artist can go about literally awake—his eyes open and his hands active—and yet dream the dreams of art ? My answer must be that it is because of his medium—for the poet, sonorous words ; for the sculptor, marble ; or for the builder, stone. It is the artist's medium that keeps him unconscious. The sculptor, if it were not because he is continually mesmerised by clay or marble, would wake up and become the mere vulgar deviser of commonplace shapes. The presence of marble and a chisel keeps him asleep.

Nowhere is the doctrinaire aloofness of the philosophical writers on æsthetic so exasperating as just at this point. They either say that *à priori* there can be no such thing as medium, or else they ignore it altogether. But the problem of medium is the key to the problem of art. If only writers of philosophical aesthetic could be induced to write nursery rhymes or play the piano !

Bosanquet, with all his excess of logic, and his otherwise tremendous and terrifying attempts to reduce art to logical coherence, is fully aware of the significance and importance of this problem of medium. For reflective thinking such as his, it must offer an extremely difficult problem, and perhaps, therefore, the more significance attaches to his recognition of it.

This, then, would be my approach to the analysis or the interpretation of the concept of medium in art :— Medium is what keeps the artist unconscious or what induces the sleep necessary towards his creative power. It is, somehow, the contact of the artist with the earth—with the sort of dark, earthly, earthy things that have never awakened and that infect him with the power of their slumbers. The simple, primitive instance seems to me ' clay in the hands of the potter.' It is just the cool, moist, earthy feel of the clay that induces him to squeeze it and caress it and mould it ; and to forget about all the other things that have no interest compared to clay.

At the very least, medium is one of the things that distinguishes an ordinary dream of natural sleep from the dream of art. Sometimes I incline to the view that it is *the* distinction : and that the creative artist differs from the dreamer only in so far as he handles his medium. Of this much I am sure, that there is something earthly and earthy about art— something that comes from the midnight depth of earth and from the lips of her slumbering.

CHAPTER II

THE NATURE AND ORIGIN OF THE IMAGINATION

How can a man be born when he is old ? Can he enter the second time into his mother's womb and be born ?
Gospel of St. John

The true meaning of propositions lies always ahead of fully conscious usage. BOSANQUET

(1)

THE previous chapter was an attempt to exhibit a parallel between the unity of the dream and an idea conceived in waking life, on the one hand, and the unity of the poem, with an idea conceived in a non-æsthetic and, in some sense, more conscious, form of experience, on the other. Now, in this parallel or analogy we have four terms—the conscious idea, the dream, the conscious idea and the poem. It is possible that the same 'conscious idea' might, under different conditions, be related either to a dream or to a poem. But of this we cannot in the meantime be sure, nor does it, for our present purpose, greatly matter. At all events, however far the analogy may take us, however profoundly we may find it possible ever to interpret a work of art by viewing it as a dream or dream-like, the two words, art and dream, cannot with truth be made absolutely to coincide in meaning. And we found that it *was* possible to differentiate between art and dream *at least* in so far as the artist, genuinely at work as an artist, must always handle something earthy—his 'medium,' clay or marble or stone. Other

39

differences there may be—countless, perhaps, for all we know at present—but this one is clear to begin with, and offers a starting point of extraordinary and, in my view, unchallengeable, definiteness.

We had thought of this earthy ' medium ' as of something that kept the artist asleep—that prevented him from becoming too entirely awake to the ordinary demands of life. For life makes all kinds of specifically non-artistic demands. We spoke, for example, of its claims upon the intellect ; of its claims upon practical common sense, or again, upon the moral consciousness. It is to these that the artist's medium renders him oblivious—with an oblivion not dissimilar to that of sleep.

Yet though not dissimilar, it is not the same. There is a difference between the deep slumbering of a weary man and the open-eyed dreaming of the poet. It might, therefore, be possible to view the earthy medium as something that kept the artist from descending right down into the motionless depth of real sleep—as a mediation, one might almost say, between mere physiological slumber and the lighter, gentler hypnosis of poetry or music.

But, further : the artist sometimes loses touch with his medium without fully waking up. It is as though the clay were not able always to exert its hypnotic influence to the full, and yet could exert it to the extent that the potter cannot quite meet the demands of the intellectual and the practical life. The hypnotic spell is very nearly, but not quite, broken. When that happens, though the potter's hands are idle, his mind is full of images that very nearly, but do not quite, take shape in clay. He has moved, for the moment, out of perfect rapport with his medium. This transitory cessation of his artistic power links him up, for the time being, with other men who have no particular artistic gift. The common man also has images in abundance ; but the power of having images and the technique of their expression stand in no necessary correlation. How are we to classify such images, or to relate them to the dream, or to art ? They are not dreams, for they belong to waking life. They are not art, for they have no shape in clay. It is at this point, I think, we need the term imagination, to include such images and at the same time, to include the images of the artist that do find expression in his medium.

While urging, then, that the image in the artist's mind, even though it be *imagined* in clay, is an utterly different thing from the image as actually expressed in clay, I think we need an inclusive term for the whole image-life of man, whether expressed in art, expressed otherwise than in art, or not expressed at all. This, I suggest, we ought to find in the word imagination. So defined it might even include the dream itself, since in fact it is exceedingly difficult to draw the line between dreaming and phantasy in general. But for the most part ' imagination ' is, by common consent, applied to those forms of phantasy that have a little more daylight in them than dreams. Again, the forms of the imagination may have a great deal in them of what looks like thought. Much philosophic writing— and that, too, the work of the greatest philosophers— is full of phantasies, of phantasies that are filled out, so to speak, with thought. Are we to include these under the imagination ? In the last resort, I think, yes—though they lie at the opposite end of the imaginative gamut from the dreams of sleep and, therefore, are not quite purely or typically imaginative. We shall do well to shelve, for the present at least, this thorny problem of philosophic phantasies. For any rigorous logic, it cannot, of course, eventually be shelved ; as is evident from the fact that upon such a writer as Lucretius, with all the majesty of his philosophical aspiration, we are moved by an unalterable instinct to bestow the laurel wreath.

(2)

What is imagination ? Whence did it come ? Does it lead anywhere, and if so, whither ?

When we try to remember anything by aid of a mental image of the thing, the image that we summon up is strangely different from the perception of the thing itself or from anything that we see or can ever see. For the image is *of something that is past.* Contrast perception by sight with the image of something remembered, and whatever likenesses or unlikenesses there may be found between the perception and the image, the latter is distinguished in an unique way by being of the past. Psychologists have sometimes made attempts to show a continuity between the image and the percept of sense. They have tried to discover a series that should begin in a percept (in which the sensational character is unmistakeable) and that should pass by gradual transitions to the memory image (where the sensational character is quite absent). This has never been done, and it has even been pronounced by one of the most scrupulous investigators to be impossible.[1] I am inclined to think that this is the correct conclusion.

The conclusion, at all events, is just one more testimony towards the mysterious and inscrutable character of memory. That we can summon up images of the past, but that these images, real as they are and sometimes intensely vivid, are of an entirely different order from the bright, sensuous

[1] Ward. *Psychological Principles,* Chap. VII., § 1

42

impressions made upon our eyes by the present objects of sense—that is wonderful. The wonder, I think, lies in the impossibility of saying where the images come from—more precisely exemplifying, as they do, the coming "out of the nowhere into here" than any other entities we know ; and, of course, the wonder challenges us, as it ought, to find out something about the hitherto inscrutable nowhere. Language is full of figurative expressions, such as "the storehouse of memory," testifying to the reality of the nowhere, and yet by the very crudeness of their spatial metaphors serving but to mock the subtlety of interest presented by the mystery.

Percept and image, then, express an antithesis of marked significance. What this significance is, is felt by psychology in its present development rather than understood. At the present moment we only begin to realise the interest and the importance that it is to have for us. To begin with, it is stating a problem rather in miniscule. Percept and image seem rather tiny entities. So they are ; and if in the last resort the contrast between them is to acquire a genuine philosophic import for us, it can only be by regarding each as centres from which we can work outwards towards something more complete and more significant. I fancy, however, that the philosophical truth implied in the contrast between the bread by which alone man shall not live and that other than bread, also a necessity of his existence, is to be apprehended and made good only by starting from this contrast between percept (or sensation) and image.

Prima facie, it is natural to suppose that in the evolution of an organism or a species, images are of later growth than percepts. An organism that only needs to see—or feel—its prey, and then to clutch it and eat it, does not appear to need the help of images. If the mere seeing and clutching did not succeed in securing the prey, the organism would perish of hunger unless it could find a new way of getting food. On such grounds one is tempted to reason that percept comes temporally before image. But at a later stage in our discussion we shall find that it is exceedingly difficult to account for seeing and touching apart from at least the *pari passu* development of images. We dare not, therefore, uncritically assert that images are of later growth than percepts.

On the other hand, when an organism cannot get food just by seeing and clutching its prey, but is compelled to devise a new way of securing food, it may very well be that such apparent biological difficulty will be beneficial to the development of the image-life of the organism—or of the species. Again, it is conceivable that in the higher animals—the human species, for example—where the image-life is well developed, such fine development of the image faculty may not be conducive to an equally fine development of the sensational powers. It is dangerous, therefore, to pre-suppose that either the power of sensation or the power of forming images is prior the one to the other.

But that danger must not prevent us from recognising the fact that when sensation and perception are in the ascendency, images are at a discount; or the correlative fact that when images are in the ascendency, perception is at a discount. In some way, difficulty in maintaining the sense-life is certainly required in order to develop the image life ; and in some way the bankruptcy of the image-life is required in order to develop sensation. In the last resort, one or the other faculties *might* be the prior. But of that we can say nothing at present.

At all events we, as human beings, do know that

44

when we cannot get what we want through direct perceptions of objects and the immediate handling of them, images arise in our mind as part of the process by which we eventually devise a way of achieving our aims. In so far as we do need to have resort to images, perception pure and simple is not enough. Though we cannot, therefore, say that images come into existence through our being forced to leave the perceptual plane of experience, we can and must say, that the development of our powers of imagery is conditioned through the impossibility of always living in perceptions and contacts.

Now what I have called the perceptual plane of experience is itself very wide. It involves all the different kinds of sensations that come through the special sense organs. It also involves all the possible combinations and inter-relations of these diverse sensations ; and when we ask how this combining and inter-relating came about, we are asking a question that probably has no answer apart from the consideration of types of experience that take us quite out of the purely perceptual. This question we must at present refrain from asking ; but it is certain that in point of fact we do find that perception in general presents an extraordinary warp and woof of all kinds of sensations. Thus perception by sight usually involves very close and complex inter-relation with perception by touch.[1]

To each special kind of sensation or perception there corresponds a special kind of images. As well as being able to hear sounds, I can also form images of sounds that I have heard ; and these sound-memories have the same strange and inscrutable difference from sounds that visual images have from the perceptions of things actually present to the eye.

---

[1] For an account of this relevant to art cf. Bereson's " tactile values " in the *Painters of the Renaissance* Series.

Further, I can also form images of sounds that I should like to hear, but have never as yet heard in my experience. Supposing it should happen to someone who is fond of music that for some reason or other he has had no opportunity of listening to music for a long time, he begins to have images of chords and melodies in his mind, and it seems probable that the dissatisfaction and restlessness that he feels through the protracted absence of the musical experience is to a large extent relieved by the images of the sounds that he summons up to himself. From considerations of this kind, let us attempt a generalisation somewhat to this effect : that when an organism is denied the satisfaction of some particular sense experience there is a tendency towards the formation of images corresponding to the particular sense which is withheld from its legitimate innings. We should need to be careful how we applied this principle, because it might very well be that sometimes when one kind of sense gratification is absent, the organism takes refuge not in indulging in the correlative images, but in some other kind of sense experience that is accessible to it. Still, if we do find cases where absence of satisfaction in sense leads to formation of corresponding images, we should not fail to note its significance.

For example, there is one kind of sense experience, the absence of which for any length of time imperils the very existence of the organism. If we are dealing with organisms where the power of image-forming corresponding to the various senses is developed in a definite and unmistakeable way, we may suppose that the images evoked through the experience of hunger will have a certain character and significance, that if not unique are at least worth special consideration. If, further, the hunger is of such a kind and so long drawn out that the existence of the organism is at stake, we do in point of fact find that the images begotten thus *in articulo mortis* have a significance that admits of no evasion of the biological question which they ask.

We might, I think, at the present stage of our argument, generalise for ourselves the antithesis between sensation and image in the words of an ancient Hebrew prophet—words as psychologically accurate and significant as anything that with all our science we could formulate to-day :—" It shall even be as when an hungry man dreameth, and, behold, he eateth ; but he awaketh and his soul is empty."[1]

We saw that one fundamental difference between image and percept is that the image is something *revived* by memory and is of the past. It is true that in speaking of the musician's power to have images in sound, these images could be rather such as he would like to hear than such as he had already heard. But then, had he never heard music at all, he could not have images of music, even of the anticipatory or creative kind. Even the novel and creative images are dependent for their peculiar character on previous, and completely past, experience of music. Yet the experience must have vanished in its entirety before it be recalled either as a memory or serve as a basis for the new, creative form of image.

> Music, when soft voices die,
> Vibrates in the memory—

but *in the memory* only after the voices have entirely died.

Clearly, then, our cue as to the nature of images lies in the fact of their being, in some sense, or to some extent, *of the past*. I am inclined to think that this is characteristic of all images whatsoever, and

[1] Isaiah, xxix., 8.

47

without any exception. On the other hand, we thought a moment ago that the musician in his images of sounds tends rather towards the imagination of sounds that he would like to hear than towards those which merely repeat his musical experience of the past. Then, too, it is clear that a great deal of our visual imagery is of things that we should like to happen to us This is the characteristic of what is generally called phantasy.. We may very naturally ask, therefore, is not all imagery as well as being stamped with the character of the past also directed towards a possible future ? One might, I think, answer unhesitatingly that a very great deal of our imagery is so directed. Whether one could go the length of saying that imagery as such is necessarily directed towards future possibilities, is another matter. In the absence of evidence to the contrary, we can only suspend judgment.

Imagination is, however, a wider term than image, and while it includes image in the narrowest and most restricted sense, it also includes the apparent thinking by which phantasy so often proceeds, no less than the emotional concomitants of all these. As imagination becomes typically imagination, the more it is directed towards possibilities and the future, the less it becomes a mere reproduction of the past.

In the imagination, therefore, we find a very curious bivalence. In form, it goes back to the past ; in direction, it seeks the future.

Imagination is then in any case stamped with the character of the past. This proposition, of course, would naturally be taken to mean the individual past of the person who imagines. The question is, however, can we so limit the term past in this relation ? We shall see. But at all events, the proposition is true, even if we do so limit it.

There are, however, many stages and many varying

kinds of experience in the life history of a man, and his imagination may bear the character of any or all of these stages. It may bear the character, for example, of what belongs to childhood. And in relation to art, at all events, the memories of childhood may be extremely important, as, for example, in a very striking way, in the poet Wordsworth. He says that his early childhood had

the glory and the freshness of a dream.

This, if literally true, is of wonderful interest. In any case, it has a curious significance for our subject.

But go far enough back, and there is found the period of early infancy of which no memories are possible. There is a period in the life history of us all which is not accessible to our individual recollection. Yet this unremembered time must have been of intense interest, and it may be extremely important, notwithstanding its having passed into oblivion.

Is there no means of finding out how our experience in childhood is related to our experience now—no way, I mean, of a more intimate kind than through merely being told about ourselves when we were babies ?

(3)

It is here that we begin to define for ourselves, and for the purposes of our discussion, the point at which the psychological investigations that issued in what is known as the psycho-analytic movement took sufficient form and character to be clearly related to the problem of art. I should hazard the view that the point in question is the discovery of the hitherto unsuspected relation that exists between early childhood and the later phases of adolescence, youth and manhood. When one thinks of Wordsworth and the *Ode on Immortality* in the light of this discovery, terms like childhood, man and boy, take on a curious new significance, call it psychological or humanistic as you please. I think there is something in the nature of a universal human truth in saying that analytical psychology relates infancy, youth and manhood in a way they never before were related. Consequently the psycho-analytic movement begins to be humanly important at the moment when, and to the extent that it can exhibit this relation.

So far as I know, there is no one who shares with Freud the honour of discovering the inner nature of the relation of the child to the mother, and of the wonderful way in which this relation continues and develops in human psychology. He found reason to suppose that underlying the closeness of the bond between mother and child, there exists in infancy on the part of the child a certain specific motive or tendency which he described as a wish—the wish, namely, for re-entrance into the comfort and security of the mother's womb. But this wish or tendency survives the period of infancy in an altogether unsuspected form ; changing the mode in which it could be expressed, no doubt ; but nevertheless persisting in some way through childhood, adolescence and maturity, and moulding the psychical history of the individual until death. In the detection of this primitive and deep-lying tendency, and in the exposition of the various modes in which it operates, Freud has shown, by common consent, the insight of genius ; and however his work is to be viewed in the light of subsequent controversy, there remains something attributable to Freud and to Freud alone, the discovery of a fact or system of psychological fact, that stands beyond all possibility of scepticism. I am not saying this as if Freud needed praise. What I am trying to do in this and what follows is to show that his discovery has an incidence upon human life and its interests as simple, natural and vital as things like food and sleep and poetry and sunlight.

But the wish or tendency towards re-entrance into the womb could never, not even in the earliest phases of childhood accessible to adult recall, express itself just as that wish or tendency. It would, so Freud conceived, always veil itself in some way. Such a veiling of the primitive instinct would be necssary and inevitable as soon as the child had any kind of independent adaptation to life. And it is, in this veiling of the primal tendency or in the changing form which it would undergo, that must be found the origin of phantasy, imagination and dream. Granted that the primitive wish does live on in some form, all the various modifications of phantasy incident to the various stages of human development would become explicable as successive modifications of it, as successive garments, so to speak, in which it would clothe, veil or disguise itself. As the growing child had to conform more and more to the social usage imposed upon it from without, the primitive tendency—or tendencies of a like primitive nature developing from it—would be more and more remote from possibility of gratification, and so would have more completely to be concealed and buried under the successive folds of symbolic imagery. In especial, the dream and its phantastic and otherwise in-explicable imagery becomes capable of explanation along the line of such a view. The dream, for Freud, is essentially a veiled desire.

Not only individual phantasy, but also those forms of the imagination which find expression in social usage and in social institutions like religion and material art are explained in the same way. They are but individual phantasies generalised, or accepted by others besides their originator. The religious *motif* of re-birth, for example, could be explained as the desire for re-entrance into the womb and re-birth under happier conditions. And here, whatever view may be taken as to the adequacy or inadequacy of Freud's explanation of religious phenomena, there can be no question as to the relevance of his science upon this most central and universal religious myth. "Except a man be born again. . . ." Does Freud explain this world-old demand of religion ? Whether or not, he certainly says something of the most supreme and vital relevance.

The Nicodemus myth is perhaps the simplest, clearest and most central instance of the application of the new science to the explanation of religious phenomena. But almost as direct is its application to the Oedipus legend in Greek tradition. The mysterious attribution of guilt to Oedipus as in the Sophocles rendering of the story really is justified psychologically. The catastrophe is not an accident of fate, but a self-inflicted punishment, an admitted retribution. Oedipus blinds himself in a real sense of guilt. When the chorus tells him it were better to be with the dead than to live sightless, he says in protest,

" Tell me not, neither counsel ye me that what is done is not most fairly done. For I know not with what gaze I could have entered Hades and looked upon my father and upon my wretched mother, since against these twain I wrought things harder to be atoned for than by the death of hanging." [1]

The guilt Oedipus feels, Freud would have said, was psychologically real ; the will to incest *was* there all the time though unrecognised.

Just as the words of Christ to Nicodemus can be related back to the fundamental desire for re-entrance into the womb, or the Oedipus myth to the unadmitted

[1] Sophocles, *Oedipus Tyrannus*, 1369-1374.

desire for incestuous union with the mother, just so—or at least on an analagous principle—all the symbolical content of religion could be traced back to such universal, primitive, psychological tendencies.

I have chosen these two illustrations—the Oedipus legend and the Nicodemus incident—first because continual reference has been made to them by all schools of analytical psychologists. These two myths serve almost as types. In the second place I have chosen them because one has a specifically artistic setting in what ranks as one of the very greatest works of literary art in antiquity ; while the other involves as typically a religious myth as it is possible to find, and one, too, that is prominent in the great historical religion of Western Europe.

I do this of set purpose. For while we do not as yet know what the relation of art to religion may turn out to be, we may not fail to remark how significant it is that illustrations taken from art and illustrations taken from religion are found side by side in the works of all the main representatives of the analytic movement. Then, again, it is to be observed that while the *Oedipus Tyrannus* of Sophocles is one of the greatest of dramatic masterpieces, either it, the play itself, or the theme which it embodies, was an integral part of the religion and religious tradition of its time. The Nicodemus episode, on the other hand, while as recorded in the gospels it may have certain elements of beauty, cannot possibly be regarded as a work of literary art—at least, not as that alone. It is primarily religious.

In all this, Freud and his school are approaching religion and art as phenomena to be explained rather than as forms of culture that have value in and for themselves. So far indeed from regarding religion, or even art, as things of value, the tendency is to treat them as pathological. They and their phenomena are symptoms of failure—of failure in adaptation. As regards the artistic question, this impression is made in the mind of the reader to an extraordinary degree in Freud's work on Leonardo. The work of a great painter is analysed to show how pathological he was. The reader would have no inkling that the art of Leonardo might be a thing of beauty. The artist failed disastrously in his adaptation to life. The causes of this failure are shown, or supposed to be shown. That is all.

Now, though I should not instance this book on Leonardo as truly representative of Freud's insight, or indeed of the methods of his school generally, it is nevertheless in such rather futile attempts that we can find the key to the limitations of the school. The Freudian psychology may be summarised as the study of the pathological—the investigation of psychological reactions and their underlying causes that do not issue in adaptation to environment. It is the psychology of mal-adaptation from the biological point of view.

The dream, if it be a veiled wish, is also an ungratified wish—a wish that never can be gratified. It is thus essentially a symptom of failure. We envisaged the whole problem of the imagination through the antithesis of percept *versus* image. Where perception —or, more generally, sensation of any kind—takes place freely and without let or hindrance there is no need for images. Images arise when we cannot perceive or cannot effect an immediate sensational contact. There would be a good case, then, for viewing images—of whatsoever kind—as indicating sensational or perceptual failure. When I cannot find something where I expected immediately to perceive it, I begin summoning up images. I do this quite involuntarily. If I were never to get beyond images, I should, so far forth be quite bankrupt in the situation. The phantasy is an image or an image system that seems to typify this remoteness from the real, tangible situation. It is as such that Freud takes it. The dream would be that image or combination of images that lay furthest from the reality of sense. In so far, then, as sensation and immediate perception are to be taken as biological success, image, phantasy and dream are to be taken as biological failure or its symptom.

This involves a negative attitude towards the imagination. The artistic imagination of Leonardo was analysed under the conception that it was an aberration and a mal-adaptation. The analysis of Leonardo's work given by Freud is, as I pointed out, an extreme case, and does not do justice to his school. But the attitude shown towards the imagination in this book is not in essentials different from the attitude shown by the whole Freudian school to the imaginative content of religion and art generally. This is not in accordance with the deep general human feeling that these things have value ; and apart altogether from the appearance of imagination in religion, the term imagination is, for mankind generally, not one of reproach, but of praise. It is only in a few phrases of satyric import that humanity has ever, I think, used the word imagination as implying blame. Its universal import is that of value.

Now failure—of whatever kind, whether biological or otherwise—is *ipso facto* not valuable. If, therefore, the general attitude of a whole school of psychologists is a tendency to regard the imagination in its various forms as symptomatic only of failure, how are we to deal with it ? With all its originality, and taking into account all our debts to it, we continue with the generality of mankind to place our emphasis upon the value or, at all events, the potential value of the imagination. It is not likely that mankind is wrong

55

here ; nor does there seem to me any doubt that its conviction has a sound psychological justification not given in the Freudian school.

But this dominant limitation of the school is also to be regarded as the limitation of a movement only at its beginning. The movement begins in relating with a certain precision childhood and infancy to manhood and adolescence. It attempts to go back to the beginnings of psychical life in so far as these can be viewed in the life of a single individual human organism. This at once raises the question, where does individual human life begin ? If we begin only at birth, we have immediately to ask, why not before birth ? If we begin with the pre-natal life, what about the whole difficult question of psychical inheritance. The Freudian school has, from the purely psychological point of view, very definitely limited itself to the single individual life history. This hesitation is bound up with that other limitation we have just discussed, under which the imaginative life is viewed as failure in biological adaptation. We shall see how these two limitations in view are correlated.

(4)

The subsequent development of the movement turns, in essentials, round the question of values. No doubt every value is in question. But for our purpose we may make the issue turn upon the value of the imagination, and the dissatisfaction that might be felt with the negative attitude of the Freudian school to this value.

The psycho-analytic movement has become a complex and many-sided thing, beset with controversy, and difficult to hold in any kind of orderly review. I think that a correct general reading of its subsequent history can nevertheless be given. A conception of its development sufficiently comprehensive to include all its aspects and embrace its many issues can, it seems to me, be found in the idea of value, or potential value, as applying to the imagination in the most general sense.

It is in the light of this general principle that we should try to approach the several particular problems as they present themselves.

What Freud did was to take the work of art, or the religious myth, and relate it according to his science of psychology, to the fundamental psychological relation of the child to the mother. He thus ' explained ' the work of art or the myth of religion. In so doing, he manifestly showed a tendency not only to explain, but to explain away. The very concepts ' art,' ' religion ' evaporated—or seemed to evaporate—as he reduced their content ever and ever more to the psychological tendency of infancy. He supposed, perhaps, that when he had shown scientifically, or from the point of view of causal sequence, the basis of the religious *motif* of re-birth, " Except a man be born again," he had done everything, in theory at least, that there was to do. But had he done everything there was to do ?

When, for example, you *know* that the story of Nicodemus coming to Jesus by night is certainly based upon a psychological characteristic universal in the life of all mankind and even now operative in your own psychology, does it follow from that indubitable knowledge, that you cease to be religious ? Does it follow that you cease to avail yourself of the religious value of the myth of re-birth ? All I should at present say is, that it does not follow.

This question, or something like this question, had a formulation or a tentative formulation, first of all,

ART AND THE UNCONSCIOUS

by Jung, in *The Psychology of the Unconscious.*[1]   In this work, it is shown how the mythology and the theological or philosophical content of a religion are related to the primitive and universal tendencies and strivings of the developing psyche. Accepting Freud's view, that in some way a tendency towards, or a desire for, return to the womb is a universal fact of infantile psychology, Jung had shown further that this desire, repressed as it must be, assumes all sorts of different forms and that these forms, as well as expressing themselves as individual phantasies, find permanent embodiment in the myths of religion or in the works of a nation's art.   So far there is but little difference from Freud, though a certain distinctive and individual manner of viewing the phenomena in question begins to make itself apparent.   The author's standpoint is, on the whole, ostensibly one which more or less judiciously considers religion as a phenomenon to be examined rather than as an experience to be lived.   It is not quite clear, however, whether Jung means the term religion, with the value that it implies, to be reserved for the religions of history ; or whether he would wish the term to be retained as possible of application to our own experience in the present in so far as it should be possible for us, in the fullest consciousness of the nature of the ' unconscious ' processes, to avail ourselves of these very processes towards the realisation of our conscious values. Perhaps the text of the book scarcely admits of this reading ; but there is implied something that leads in this direction.

As a scientist and with the aloofness of one who holds himself above the events he keeps in review, Jung does not explicitly do more than speak of religion

[1] *The Psychology of the Unconscious.*   A Study of the Transformations and Symbolisms of the Libido.   A Contribution to the History of Evolution and Thought.

as a matter of historical fact—here, a social phenomenon, there, a phenomenon of individual psychology.
He speaks, certainly, of religious symbolism as something to be escaped from, a mere bondage, in so far
as there is belief in the concrete reality of the symbol.
The idea of God, that is to say, or of the gods, is such a
bondage in so far as it is supposed that God exists
or that there are gods. But the developing human
soul must certainly produce ' unconscious ' phantasies. The psychical life-energy of man goes on
continuously transforming itself into some expression
of such phantasies, typically say, the mythological
content of religions. The primal desire for re-
entrance to the womb, never expressing itself nakedly,
but veiling itself as Freud had supposed under all
kinds of symbolism, gives us in this very symbolism
what history has called religion.

It is at this point that sense of value in the imagination begins to make itself felt, and even to be definitely
asserted by the writer. The extraordinary modifications and transformations of the original infantile
desire were, for primitive races, as well as inevitable,
also necessary. On the lowest grounds, they would
afford scope for an otherwise baneful manifestation of
the life energy. But the new point of view that
emerges in the latter part of *The Psychology of the
Unconscious* discovers in this religious symbolism
other possible functions—less negative than the mere
absorption or transformation of a dangerous energy.
The embodiment of individual phantasy and racial
myth in works of art and in ceremonies and monu-
ments of religion has given us things of " imperishable
beauty." Now that is a value, a positive value, and
not a mere safeguard, not just a sublimation of
destructive force.

From the point of view of a theory of art this, of
course, is an all-important admission. It gives us

59

the fundamental principal of which we are in search. To utilise that principle, however, in its full bearing, we need to follow the writer of *The Psychology of the Unconscious* in a further development of his subject.

The idea to which he is introducing us is that the lines of action leading to another stage of social or individual development were indicated by these religious phantasies ; or at least that it was through these phantasies, and by their aid, that the higher stage was reached.

This new conception of the import of phantasy gives us a means of understanding the religious consciousness such as Western Europe, at least, has not had along the lines of scientific and reflective thought.

Something of the kind may have been done before or elsewhere symbolically or intuitively. Of this I cannot speak. But in terms of Western Science, this conception of Jung's has such a penetrating incidence on the problem of religion and so challenges all other contemporary efforts towards a philosophy of religion, that we must allow ourselves some rein for its discussion.

When Freud stresses that aspect of the ' unconscious ' process in which the real intention is concealed in an elaborate disguise, it is stated, implied or taken for granted, that primitive, infantile wishes do operate as such. In a phenomenology of ' the unconscious ' like Jung's *Psychology of the Unconscious* where the accent of interest is thrown over on to the variety, strangeness, beauty, ugliness, apparent relevance or irrelevance of the imagery with which the initial *motif* is clothed, it becomes natural to ask for the significance of all that variety and strangeness : If it is sometimes beautiful, wherefore the beauty ? If it is sometimes apparently relevant to new issues, wherefore that relevance ? If to all appearance irrelevant, wherefore so arbitrary ?

Again, if primitive or infantile desires, such as that for re-entrance into the womb, be seriously brought up to adult psychology for comparison, can it be true to say that the full-grown man does really cherish the desire of incest, unacknowledged, or unknown to himself ? On the other hand, if a phantasy like that of desire for re-birth, be taken as the religious consciousness takes it—as a desire, that is to say, for a new and better orientation to life, does not this reading at once state a true fact about the psychology of the man and at the same time *preserve* all that is true and vital in Freud's original contention ?

There is another and more positive aspect of this reading of the matter. In the symbolism by ' the unconscious ' of the relationship between the son and the mother there appear tentative efforts through which the baneful tie might be broken. The primitive symbolism of the unconscious shows not only the *motif* of re-birth, but the direction in which re-birth is to take place, and the means of its accomplishment, if it is to be successful and effective. There is " a battle for deliverance from the mother "[1] in which the fighter is aided and led on from point to point by the multitudinous detail of the imagery that indicates his pathway.

Now in the past—in the days of any of the great historical religions at their best—such religious symbolism would operate unconsciously, in this sense, that the primitive religious mind could not be aware of the nature and origin of the symbolism of which it availed itself. Action might be based upon symbolism, or be fruitful through the effective use of symbolism ; and so far as this might be the case, religion, in the past at all events, would have its own value.

[1] The title of Chapter VI. in *The Psychology of the Unconscious*.

But the secret of the origin of phantasy was, of course, not in the possession of the primitive religious mind. In that sense, or to that extent, it might correctly be called unconscious.

Any such unconscious following of the symbolising instinct must, however, be incompatible with our modern scientific standpoint. We have now a higher degree of consciousness of the inner mode of working of ' the unconscious ' ; and we cannot therefore allow ourselves any longer blindly to follow the lead of the symbolising instinct. On the other hand, we know that the developing psychical life of man *will* always go on producing phantasies. What we can do, therefore, is consciously to recognise this ; and to avail ourselves of the fact, if we may. In the past it had been simply religion which had enabled men to use their phantasy life " as a bridge " to all their greatest achievements. In religion they did this without fully knowing what they were doing, and their success was independent, not perhaps of any conscious intention, but certainly independent of the real knowledge of the imaginative processes and their origin, which in the nature of the case, they could not have possessed. We, in our full consciousness of the nature of our imagination, have lost both the power and the right thus to follow any merely instinctive and unknowing path to achievement. For us now at the present day, it is only through conscious recognition and understanding that it is possible to take possession of our own psychical energy and use it for life.

Would the author of *The Psychology of the Unconscious* at this stage in his thinking have called such a standpoint the religious one ? This, I suggested, is a matter perhaps not quite clearly articulated. For he speaks as if we could take possession of the psychical energy " bound up in incest," though it does not with definiteness appear whether or not we any longer need religion or a religious faith for this end. " This," he says, " would be the course of moral autonomy, of perfect freedom, when man could without compulsion wish that which he must do and this from knowledge without delusion through belief in the religious symbols."[1] It is clear, indeed, that we must have liberation from belief in the religious symbols of the past, but it does not clearly appear in what way the idea is to be made actual of entering into possession of our psychical energy through the conscious understanding of its unconscious workings.

What is clear is the extent to which the writer has achieved a re-valuation of the imaginative powers of mankind. Another essential aspect of " the unconscious " and its nature has, however, still to be exhibited before the idea of value can be completely related to the imagination in the totality of its range.

It is obvious how deeply *The Psychology of the Unconscious* is indebted to the mythology of past ages for its interpretation of individual psychology. Reciprocally, of course, that mythology receives its elucidation through the individual. Thus the method becomes gradually clear, through which the two aspects, the individual and the racial, can be correlated. For the individual must repeat in some way the psychology of his race. There is no difficulty in saying that it is so. The difficulty begins when we try to define how it is so, and in what way the past of his race is inherited by the individual.

It is obvious that by oral tradition and by education, if not in many more subtle ways, the individual in his personal experience from birth onwards receives into his psyche all the rich content of the recorded past that tradition and education can give. This would account to some extent, at all events, for the occur-

[1] *Psychology of the Unconscious.* Eng. translation, p. 144.

rence in dream and phantasy of material that otherwise might be supposed to belong entirely to the past. In Freud's view, or on the general grounds which he took for granted in the development of his psychological method, it was a sufficient account of all that wealth of imagery that belongs to dream and phantasy.

But the individual does inherit the qualities of his race. He has eyes and ears that come to him as his heritage from a very long line of evolution, and he is in possession of the smooth and unhindered mechanism of those organs by which sight and hearing are possible and effective. No one disputes this. He has also brain and nerves, they also rendered effective in their working by the preceding ages of their evolution and use. Has he not also an inheritance from the past of which an account could be given in more specifically psychological terms ? Plato used to speak of reminiscence—of the remembering by the soul of its experience before the birth of the body. Philosophy used to be cognizant of a controversy about innate ideas. Can ideas be inherited ? Neither the idiom of Plato, nor that of Descartes and Leibniz is one which has any special appeal to us now. Our modern science has discarded that idiom or denuded it of its significance. Nevertheless the old question returns in a new form. What *psychological* account have we to give of our inheritance from the past of our race ?

The dreams of all have a certain similarity of structure and community of content. Individuals living together in the same society no doubt have a common experience which enters into their dreams. But this individual or personal experience is not of itself sufficient to explain the peculiar form and material of the dream. At the very outset, it does not explain the irrational and unintelligible character of the dream, its discordance with the real conditions of present life. This is, however, a universal character and one universally admitted.

The same chaotic, irrational and unreal character belongs to archaic myths ; and from the point of view of the culture of civilised races it belongs also to the psychology of primitive and savage tribes. That the dream is an archaic form of consciousness, partaking in a high degree the character of the consciousness of the primitive, and re-asserting itself under the conditions of sleep, is a hypothesis which accords admirably with all the psychological data in question and renders them intelligible in a way that no other hypothesis has done.

The formulation which Jung gave to this view was through the category of archetypal image. Just as instinct is an inherited mode of action *vis-a-vis* a certain type of object, so the archetypal image is to be regarded as the inherited mode of psychical apprehension of the object. Instinct has always been known and admitted as a matter of external observation. Its psychical counterpart has not received recognition. It is of this correlative, however, that we have so pressing a need to give some genuinely psychological account. The archaic image or archetype, then, is the term used to denote those images or image systems which are not derived from personal experience, but which are inherited from the racial past.

It is easy to see, on the one hand, how organs like eyes and ears, brain and nerve, are inherited, or at all events easy to admit that they *are* inherited ; and it is also easy to see, on the other, how the past of the race is inherited through culture and education and by all the subtle means of communication that one human being has with another, and very especially and subtly, parent with child. It is not so easy to admit that images or ideas, in any sense as images and ideas, can be inherited. This, however, is the proposition which challenges us, and which we have carefully to lay before us and examine. It is, I think, to be understood, as a *via media* between the concept of mere physiological inheritance, on the one hand, and that of inheritance by oral tradition, on the other, even in its most subtle and unconscious forms.

Too long our culture has been content to build its structures upon ideas of physiological transmission on the one hand and upon ideas of history and tradition on the other. Both ways of viewing the transmission are real enough, but until the significance and the vitality of the idea of psychical or psychological continuity is realised and utilised, there will remain in our culture a barrenness and sterility from the disability of which we cannot free ourselves.

In *The Psychology of the Unconscious*, the new idea is implicit and germinating. One of the most beautiful forms of this germination is a little passage on a poem of Nietzsche, where it is said, " That which in Nietzsche appears as a practical figure of speech is really a primitive myth. It is as if the poet still possessed a dim idea or capacity to feel and re-activate those imperishable phantoms of long-past worlds of thought in the words of our present-day speech and in the images which crowd themselves into his phantasy." This sentence may perhaps be taken to typify or summarise the attitude of Jung to the problem in *The Psychology of the Unconscious*.

Before passing on to later formulations of the idea of the archetype, it might be well to ask how, for our present purpose, we could best illustrate what is meant by an archaic image. It has always seemed to me that, for purposes of general psychological formulation, the idea or image of the mother is by far the best and by far the least open to criticism. Jung instances the idea of God, for example, and the idea of energy

66

as also dominant and inherited *motifs* in all human psychology. I believe they are ; and in passing I cannot help observing how continually present these *motifs* are in the art of the whole world, and how they lend themselves to transfiguration in the beauty of art and literature. But I cannot help thinking at the same time that they exhibit the fundamental psychological principle of which we are in search with far less clearness and security than does the image of the mother. The latter, too, has this advantage, that it enables us at every point to compare the later development of analytic views with the original Freudian discovery, of the relation of child to mother, and so to formulate precisely the essential differences in the conceptions of the several schools.

For while the image or archetype of the mother is universally present in human psychology, it cannot either fully be described or explained in terms of the experience—*i.e.*, the experiencing by the individual—of the actual mother, or in terms of any individual experience whatsoever. It is essentially archaic in structure and not deducible, in its entirety, from the individual experience as given through the social or cultural conditions of the present. The phrase, " collective unconscious," is the formula through which Jung summarises the totality of such archetypal images and their inter-relation. The force of the term, collective, lies in the emphasis placed upon repetition in racial experience of situations that must, in the nature of the case, be of universal and never-ceasing occurrence in the history of the evolution of the human organism, and whose traces are, therefore, found in the psychology of all men.

An initial view of the conception of this hereditary factor in experience can, I think, best be given in Jung's own words, by placing together two concise observations made with respect to it. In the first

(1917) he says, " The absolute or collective unconscious contains the inherited world-images generally, under the form of primordial images or mythological themes."[1] In the second (1922) he speaks as if with a certain kind of reservation, or wish to correct a possible misconception : " In itself, the collective unconscious cannot be said to exist at all ; that is to say, it is nothing but a possibility, that possibility, in fact, which from primordial time has found expression in the definite form of mnemic images or anatomical structure. It is inherited in the structure of the brain. It does not yield inborn ideas, but inborn possibilities of ideas."[2]

The first of the two passages, if it does not actually fall nearer the truth, has a certain suggestiveness that the second does not contain. The matter does not seem in any essential philosophical respect different from the old controversy about innate ideas. The first citation may, if the reader choose, be taken to err in the direction of making the inherited material an image in a too literal sense of the term ; the second certainly does err in the direction of restricting the inheritance too entirely to a potentiality. Whenever you overstress one side of the matter by speaking of innate ideas in all their full-fledged dignity as ideas, you will always find a complacent little Locke emerging ' out of the unconscious ' ready to answer you " in one word, by experience." Whenever you overstress the other side of the matter and whittle your terminology down to the merely " inborn possibility of ideas," you will always be confronted by a discontented little Leibniz with the remark, " Les puissances véritables ne sont jamais de simples possibilités." If, therefore, we cannot accept the first mode of statement in its

[1] *Analytical Psychology.* Eng. translation, p. 438.
[2] *On the Relation of Analytical Psychology to Poetic Art.* British Journal of Psychology, Medical Section, 1923, Vol. III., Part 2, pp. 228, 229.

literalness, we must not lose sight of its peculiar suggestiveness, and of the novelty of its psychological implications.

The formulation, however, that seems to me most satisfying and most nearly to hold the balance between these two extremes, is that given towards the end of *Psychological Types*.[1] " These archetypes, whose *innermost nature is inaccessible to experience,* represent the deposit of psychic functioning of the whole ancestral line, *i.e.*, the heaped-up, or pooled, experiences of organic existence in general, a million times repeated, and condensed into types. Hence, in these archetypes, all experiences are represented which since primeval times have happened on this planet. Their archetypal distinctness is the more marked, the more frequently and intensely they have been experienced. The archetype would be—to borrow from Kant—the noumenon of the image which intuition perceives and, in *perceiving, creates.*"

The italics are mine, and the italicised words bring out the precise difficulty involved, viz., that the innermost nature of the archetype is inaccessible to experience *and yet* that it—or any manifestation of it—is created only in experience.

Perhaps we have not really got further than this negative point of view that there is a factor in human experience that is neither given or accounted for by the personal experience of the individual from birth nor yet that can be stated in terms of physiological transmission. But if we hold fast even to this negative statement, we shall have sufficient to go upon so far as the nature of art is concerned in relation to the past experience of the race.

[1] *Psychological Types, or the Psychology of Individuation.* Eng. translation, pp. 507, 508.

ART AND THE UNCONSCIOUS

(5)

And now, when we return to art, it seems almost needless to point out how the archaic appears both in the things that are presented to our sense and in the mode of that presentation. Poetry tells you about things that have happened long ago, and it tells you about them in language that is rich with an antique idiom. It seems to me very simple and quite true to say that both in form and content poetry is archaic. But if I am met with the old objection that in art there is no distinction between content and form, I am satisfied with saying that it uses every artifice and exerts all its powers to take you back into past phases of experience and into the ancient history of peoples.

As well as to the racial past, equally and *pari passu*, the poet takes you back into his own individual past. The poet must, I think, be regarded as striving after the simplicity of a childish utterance. His goal is to think as a child, to understand as a child. He must deliver himself—and the poetic task is the same in every age—from the burden of the intellect of his day and the complexity of the forms of speech which it involves.

Thus with the simplicity of utterance which Milton viewed as one of the essentials of poetry, there is bound up also the poet's own childhood, and its memories of which he is trying to catch a glimpse. In that poem, where of all others, the childish experience is most intimately in question, it is the poet's own childhood, which he is trying to recall. No doubt Wordsworth would be the high court of appeal if we wanted evidence of the presence of more than an individual past. But the individual past is presented with simplicity and is to be taken as the first reality. It is indeed through that extraordinary simplicity in the reference to " the splendour in the grass, the glory in the flower," that I try to explain to myself the beauty of the language ; but you could not find it so simple if you took it otherwise than just about his own real childhood. The way in which these two childhoods, then, the individual childhood and the childhood of the race, are blended and mingled will vary from poem to poem ; and it need not be apparent on the surface how much of either is present. Both are always there. The mere fact of verse and rhythm would be enough to prove that.

"Hush-a-bye baby on the tree top. . . ."

That is the kind of experience to which the poet is always reverting.

Here we should have to observe that every artistic tradition carries with it this love of the past to such an overwhelming extent that it becomes almost a touchstone of individual genius whether it can find the past that belongs to it and to which alone it has any right.

The tale of Troy is for ever divine, but not every poet need sing of Troy. Of what past, then, shall he sing, and in what kind of antique idiom ? It is for his own genius to decide. When he has written, and the work is good, the measure of his genuis is the depth to which he has gone back, the originality of his idiom the degree of its antiquity. Or in other words, his genius must lead him to those recollections of an ancient world where his ' archetypal ' inheritance will most entirely sustain and reinforce his ' traditional ' inheritance. When Keats is able to hear, and once more to articulate, that " large utterance of the early gods," it is because the burden of the antique pressed upon him not only from the outside and by way of the studious enrichment of his experience, but also because the antique spirit burdened him from within and by way of a peculiarly strong inheritance of that spirit in its ' archetypal ' form. *Hyperion* would have given him deliverance from the burden had he been able more completely to effect the union of the inner inheritance with the external forms of his experience. The harmonisation of the inner with the outer thus becomes at least one of the formulæ through which we can have some access to the secret of poetic genius.

The admission of the archaic, then, in art is essential to the understanding of its nature. But the imagination is something more than the material of art. Art is only one of the goals to which it may lead. The more general principle is that so far as the archaic can be recognised and made integral with individual and social experience it necessarily gives an enlargement and enrichment of these experiences. If, in the language of *The Psychology of the Unconscious* its presence in art has given us things of " imperishable beauty from the æsthetic standpoint," this doubtless gives us a type of its transformation that can be read with peculiar ease and clearness.

But if the transformation and assimilation of the archaic in religion is the wider and more inclusive principle, we cannot even for the purpose of æsthetic, limit our consideration to the æsthetic problem alone. For we do not as yet know how the archaic becomes transfigured in art, whether directly through a direct and immediate artistic impulse, or whether mediately, through religion. Quite conceivably it undergoes transformation in art in both ways—both directly and indirectly. On the other side, too, on the side of the completed and permanent beauty of art, we do not know where the value of that beauty may lie. Does it lie in the presence of beauty as something enjoyed entirely for its own sake and valuable exclusively in the act of enjoyment ? Or does it lie in some subtle power that art may have of causing a kind of paradoxical discontent with its own beauty and urging the people who enjoy it to go on into spheres of life that lie beyond art and have values other than those of beauty. Perhaps, again both. At all events, these are questions that emerge, difficult but inevitable.

Now, if the value of art, or any other value, be conditioned through our racial inheritance in the sense above defined, there is involved also the idea of plasticity in the archaic images or in their expressions in individual experience. That is why the attitude towards the archaic becomes the touchstone separating the various schools of psychology. It is a question of the plasticity of the inherited psychical material The archetype can receive its expression in individual experience in one way rather than in another. There is a possibility of choice. This brings us to the fundamental problem of ethics—that of freedom. With such an immense and difficult problem we cannot, of course, be concerned here. But for my own part I am bound to say it is quite as unacceptable to regard art as the automatic product of brain and nerves as it is to regard the human being as an automaton in the sphere of conduct. And whatever view is taken of ethical freedom or of creativeness in art, plasticity of psychical material is an essential for the reality of these conceptions in any sense, or from any standpoint.

(6)

This brings me to the final topic in my exposition of what I conceive to be the origin and nature of the imagination. It is the question as to the mode in which the primitive or crude material of the imagination can be made available for life. The term, symbol, has been freely used during the growth of the analytic movement, but the sense in which it has been employed by Jung will require special consideration. He regards a symbol as an expression for that of which no rational account can be given at the time when the symbol possesses its highest value. It is thus an indication of the future, of the general direction which life, individual or social, must follow. At a later date, or for a generation for whom a certain symbol has ceased to be vital, it may be possible to find another expression—as for example, an intelligible account—of what the symbol originally implied or indicated. But in so far as any kind of additional expression becomes possible, it means that the symbol has already been so far forth devitalised. The example which Jung gives and which seems to me to epitomise his intention with a peculiar force and significance is that of the Christian Cross. " The way in which St. Paul and the early mystical speculators handle the symbol of the Cross shows that for them it was a living symbol which represented the inexpressible in an *unsurpassable way.*"[1]

The reproach of mysticism brought against the originator of this view of symbolism is familiar enough. The term, symbol, however stands at once in contemporary psychological literature for an idea of which some intelligible account has to be given, and also in religion and art for an idea that must be made concrete, and rendered available for the purposes of criticism, of philosophy, and of culture as a whole. I admit that Jung, in accordance with his general method, writes with an extraordinary and perhaps altogether undue condensation. But in his exposition of symbolism there is for me, I feel bound to contend, no mysticism, but a certain view of teleology that is as capable of elucidation and criticism as any psycho-

[1] *Psychological Types.* Eng. translation, p. 602.

logical or philosophical doctrine can be, and subject only to the limitations that necessarily beset every attempt in these departments of thought.

The symbol is regarded as something placed over against the conscious standpoint. Or rather, the image or the phantasy, in all the fulness of its emotional resonance and with all the apparent thought-content through which it may have been elaborated, becomes a symbol through the adoption by consciousness of a definite attitude towards it. Through the symbol, or *vis-à-vis* the symbol, the conscious being commits himself, of his own choice, to a certain course of conduct, life, or experience. He does not, and cannot, fully know where he is being led ; though knowledge may grow, from more to more, as he makes good each step of the way. As he advances, the symbol will change, or the imagery involved will change. Again, the changing imagery may become symbolic afresh through the re-orientation to it of the conscious individual ; but so far as the original symbol is concerned, its significance becomes lessened as he advances ; and he may eventually reach a point where it falls altogether out of sight. Thus for many individuals, and for certain sections of society, the Christian Cross is, in this view, no longer of any but an historical significance. It has ceased to be a symbol.

The conception is thus essentially teleological in so far as the enrichment of life, or the moral individuality, is gained and secured. It is a teleology in which purpose is, at the most, implicit, in so far as no intellectual formulation of aim is, or can be, achieved. The term purpose, is, in effect misleading. For, at a later stage, what becomes explicit is not so much purpose or aim as realised value.

How, in accordance with our general method, can we bring our psychological thinking up to this view of the teleological in life ?

75

ART AND THE UNCONSCIOUS

We had regarded the development of images not necessarily as originating from, but certainly as conditioned by, a breach in the continuity of the sensational or perceptual life that every organism (or species) must sustain, more or less, if it is to survive. In so far as images just arose, just appeared and offered no cue towards a return to sensation, to the basal conditions of life like sex and nutrition, they might, we had conceived, be regarded as mere pathological phenomena. If, on the other hand, they could once more be brought up to the biological situation they offered a new means towards life, even on the sensational plane. And in so far as the successful reaction was once more secured, the images that led to it would become needless and would vanish from the life of the organism, at least for the time being, and as regards the successful orientation.

We had regarded, also, the initiation of the psychoanalytic movement as a special study of unsuccessful reactions of the human organism on the sensational plane. Symptomatic of this maladaptation, the dream played a conspicuous part. If, on the other hand, the individual could secure a new and successful biological orientation, the dream would disappear as a phenomenon of his consciousness. It is, at all events relatively, easy to see how in the case of the obtrusion of some simple image in consciousness, that image will vanish when the appropriate response is made. If I cannot find a book where I think I have put it, I may be beset—or plagued—with images of possible places in which I might hope to find it. If and when I do find it, these images automatically disappear.

It is by no means such a simple matter to obtain any kind of intuition as to the way in which the dream may vanish from a man's habitual slumbers as he tries more perfectly to adapt himself to his environment. Should we, however, attempt to subsume the two cases under one general principle ? I think so, but not before returning to an important observation already made. We saw that sensation and perception, on the one hand, are antithetical to image-formation, on the other, in so far as each type of experience must give place to the other ; but we dared not assume the priority of the one over the other. We cannot, then, at this point assume the priority of sensation to image.

If, therefore, the simple phenomena of the images in the illustration I have made use of about looking for the lost book are to be regarded as in essentials the same as the far more complex phenomena of dreams in their gradual changing and vanishing as the individual secures his completer adaptation to life, it must be done without any assumption either that sensation is prior to image or that image is prior to sensation. The claims of sensation and image, and all that the antithesis may most profoundly imply, must be investigated on their own merits and judged impartially.

With this safeguard, there seems no reason to suppose that the scrutiny of the simpler phenomena may not shed light on the more complex. In so far as one may insist on the *revived* character of all images, in so far as everything that can be called image, is, on one side, related to past experience ; and in so far as there appears to be a real continuity between individual and racial past, I am inclined closely to relate the phenomena of memory images to the phenomena of dream and phantasy. As we proceed with our study of the psychology of art, we may find many illustrations that will, I hope, serve to bring together the various aspects of memory, phantasy and dream, and to exhibit a relation between them.

So far as regards dream and phantasy we have supposed that in actual fact, the better orientation of a man to life, is co-ordinate with the disappearance of the dream, and of the phantasy, at least in a pathological aspect. When we ask for the *modus operandi* of all this, or if we demand a method whereby the process can receive the guidance of consciousness, it is obvious that there is implied *a conscious attitude of the subject* towards this phantasy or his dreams—towards the products of his imagination in the widest sense. With this implication of a conscious attitude of the subject towards his phantasy, there emerges, again, the view of phantasy as symbolical.

We are indeed very far from being able to unify and systematise the phenomena of the imagination in the way that I have suggested. In so far as it may be possible to do so, we are under no greater disabilities than those to which any psychological method is liable. Metaphysical questions, such as that of freedom, do indeed emerge ; but that difficulty would be incident to any psychology without reserve or exception.

At the least, such considerations seem to me to make it well worth while to keep in view the idea of the symbol as something that naturally expresses itself in art. Perhaps, even, the essence of art is its symbolic function.

Our starting point at the beginning of this chapter was the parallel between art and dream. There, however, it was a question of the transition from the conscious idea to the dream or to the poem. Now, in our discussion of symbolism, we return once more to the conscious point of view, but *after* the dream has been dreamed, *after* the poem has been written. In so far as we can regard dream or poem as a symbol it has now become a question of the attitude of consciousness *vis-à-vis* the work of art. We might regard it, then, as if there were a rhythm—consciousness, the unconsciousness of dreaming, return to consciousness. It is the rhythm, indeed, of day and night ; of conscious life, sleep and waking again.

Now we have not ventured entirely to identify the work of art with the symbol. We have only got the length of supposing that art may be profoundly symbolical in character. It does not seem an unwarranted assumption to say that much of the greatest art is thus symbolical. But perhaps not all art, not every type of beauty, is exclusively or essentially symbolical. At present we cannot be more than tentative.

In so far as we do feel warranted in keeping the symbolical character of art in view, it would become the middle term—the transition—between two conscious attitudes or ideas. The artist, with his intellectual or moral orientation goes off upon his artistic quest, passes into the unconsciousness of his art, and wakes up again when the finished product leaves his hand.

Just in so far as we could accept this account of the matter, just so far also would it give us a principle of differentiation between the creative and the appreciative in experience of beauty. If art be symbolic, it is the artist who discovers the symbol. But he need not—though of course he may—recoginse it as a symbol. We, the appreciative recipients of his work, must so recognise it. Or, at least, it is thrown out over against us, objectively, with all the challenge of a symbol. We may thus describe two quite different attitudes of consciousness. The first, that of the artist before the period of his creative dreaming, is clearly distinguishable from the second, that of the appreciative or critical mind confronted with the thing of beauty.

Thus, again, I see no reason for any attempt to identify, or to confuse, the creative power in art with the critical or the receptive. Art, then, is essentially social, because every artefact, however individual, is presented to many minds. And once again, we are forced back upon the importance of the concept of medium, this time as standing between and bringing together the lonely genius of the artist and the many-sidedness of social criticism and response.

For both dreaming and imagery may be absolutely lonely and incommunicable. Alike the dreamer and the day-dreamer have made their profound impression upon other minds—now of curiosity, now of pity. But the curiosity remains ungratified, and the regret cannot merge into sympathy—

> pity these have not
> Traced upon vellum of wild Indian leaf
> The shadows of melodious utterance,
> But bare of laurel they live and dream and die ;
> For Poesy alone can tell her dreams—
> With the fine spell of words alone can save
> Imagination from the sable chain
> And dumb enchantment.

Or, otherwise and reverting to the primitive idea of the clay in the potter's hands—" take up of the dust of the earth," on however small a scale, and shape it somehow, there imagination is at work and as it works it communicates itself.

For people can see you, and in this rudimentary sociability is also the germ of the constructive imagination that belongs to the greatest or most abiding or most commanding forms of art. After all, all the genuine, deep delight of life is in showing people the mud-pies you have made ; and life is at its best when we confidingly recommend our mud-pies to each other's sympathetic consideration.

We, therefore, return to the elaboration of the concept of medium with a new cue, that of sociability or communicability—the meeting of spirit with spirit. This seems to imply a curious entanglement of earthiness and spirituality. But I think that is correct. What is art but an entanglement—or perhaps rather a synthesis—of the most earthy and the most spiritual ?

CHAPTER III

PLASTICITY AND VISION

Oui, l'oeuvre sort plus belle
D'une forme au travail
Rebelle,
Vers, marbre, onyx, email.

THEOPHILE GAUTIER

A great artist who above all things delineates his object; who
subordinates expression to that which it is designed to express.

MATTHEW ARNOLD

AGAIN I must ask the reader to come with me into
a more nebulous region—a region where fine distinctions and articulate propositions are for the time
being impossible. Again we must sacrifice distinctness to our sense of massiveness, and of the larger
relations of the more massive things to each other.
We must try to appreciate general proportions before
we can arrive at clearness of outline and detail.

(1)

We saw that we could not, that we dared not,
understand the Beatrice of the *Comedia* as just
Beatrice Portinari invested with the colour and the
light of heaven. We must understand her as
essentially part of Dante himself—the part that
reveals him to himself.

If so, the reader will ask, are not all the characters
of a poem just bits of the poet—not the men and
women that he knew, but aspects of himself ? Or
more generally still, and by the same logic, are not
all stories just a rendering of the author's own history
—record of the adventures of his own soul ? If the

81

import of this question could be fully perceived we should have got a long way towards the solution of some great problems of art. For, of course, we have to make the still wider generalisation, and to ask whether all art in so far as it portrays, or appears to portray, human forms, be not simply an exposition of the artist's mind and heart, an exposition in terms that no doubt appear as the forms of his friends, but that are just in reality fragments of his own soul ? As in the case of Dante's Beatrice, it might in many other cases be possible to answer the question in the same way. Thus the lady of the pictures of Botticelli might well be taken as the subjective revealer of the secrets of *his* heart, or the Ariadne likewise for Titian, or the Madonna for the genuinely inspired among the earlier artists of the Renaissance. But there is a certain kind of story we call tragedy or comedy, a story that is supposed to be played upon the ear and before the eye of the spectator by living, moving, speaking men and women. Here also, will it not be true that the tragedy is just the conflict of the author's soul—of its expectations, its failures and its loss ? The logic of our position would compel us to say yes, were it not because of the living players themselves. In a poem like the *Comedia* the poet is free to express himself as he will, or rather, it is " the lady of his mind " who is free and who comes to the possession of her own free life as he writes. But for the tragic poet there is a difference. The actress indeed stands to him, apparently, much as the canvas and the paint stand to the painter. She seems to be part of his medium and must, at all events, repeat the words allotted to her. But then—and here is the difference—she is also his interpreter. She it is, once more, who has to reveal the poet to himself ; but the self-revealer can no longer remain a purely subjective figure or form. She is a living lady, and she

has the rights of her own life. The tragedian, therefore, is not free in the sense in which Dante is free.
He must write something which the actress may
interpret : he may only write what she *can* interpret. And here the laws and the structure and
the history of *her* own soul come in with all their
irresistible claims. She is herself part of some other—
not story, but—history, and her ability to act at all
depends upon this actual historical setting with all
her particular loves and hates, her birth race and the
tradition of her own gods.

But if she be thus an artist in her own right, our
logic would at once invite us to ask : What is the
medium of *her* art ? Obviously the medium of
dramatic art in general must include the stage and
all the stage mechanism and trappings, and perhaps
much else besides. To attempt at present fully to
define it would take us too far. In the meantime we
have only to touch upon it in so far as it concerns
the relation of the playwright and the actress. Just
looking at her on the stage as she speaks or dances,
our first thought would naturally be that she is part
of the dramatist's medium. But then, we had to
ask about medium from *her* point of view, and together with that question she appeared not only as
part of his medium, but also as his interpreter—to
his audience, no doubt, as something too obvious
to mention, but to himself also, in the last resort.
True, dramatists need not in general write for any
particular actress they know ; but they may not
write for abstractions. They must write for living
women, who are also artists.

The actress thus presents, as it were, a point of
divergence. She appears as at once the interpreter
and the medium ; but because she claims a medium
of her own, and because that claim must, of course,
be conceded, the two concepts will not quite coincide.

Now what *is* the medium of her art ? Suppose we
were to make her a dancer, or at least to place the
accent upon the choric side of her art, I think the
suggestion would emerge that the medium here is
just her own body. That, at all events, is precisely
the cue that I should wish to follow. It would also
give us what we want from the point of view of the
playwright or the chorographer. He stands *vis-à-vis*
the actress. He sees her body and just *feels* it as his
medium. So far he is almost a plastic artist, and as
such remains the master and controlling mind. But
then in so far as he intuits a spiritual individuality
behind the veil of the flesh, he makes her into the
interpreter, who is indeed one half self-revealer, but
also one half resistent and unplastic individuality.
Here he loses his mastery and acknowledges that the
creativeness of the whole show can never rest with
him alone. The two of them have, therefore, to
form a kind of society and to discover a common
purpose. In so far as they can achieve this common
purpose, they both fall back together upon the same
medium, viz., the moving body of the actress herself.

Let us go back for a moment to Athenian tragedy
and the Attic drama. It was a specifically religious
and social function. In particular, the chorus of the
Athenian tragedy gives us something of an acknow-
ledged social and religious quality never quite so
fully admitted in any other epoch of dramatic art.
In the chorus the element of historical allusion and
social tradition is overpoweringly strong. The whole
occasion of the performance of an Attic tragedy was
a religious festival ; the audience, the chorus, and
the tragic theme itself were related to each other in
ways so clearly defined that Aschylus or Sophocles
or Euripides never even thought of turning aside
from the traditionally accepted material of tragedy,
Agathon being the first to make the innovation of

an entirely new theme. In their respect they had an incomparably lower degree of freedom than the dramatist of the modern world. Since they were so limited, their tragic poetry must be something other than merely the history of their own souls. Whole masses of historical and traditional and mythological material have to enter into the fabric of their dramatic work ; and the resulting tragedy has, in large parts of it, to be sung by the chorus, which, it must be remembered, was always and essentially a dance.

There is something in the art of dancing very far removed from the inward quietness and subjectivity of the narration of a simple tale in prose or verse. Here the living and moving bodies of men and women intervene very effectually between the poet and his subjectivity. Parts of himself there must be, no doubt, in the dancers and their movements : and certainly they shall not cease, because they are dancers, to reveal the poet to himself. But in dancing, the living object through which the tragic tale is told begins to have a kind of supremacy over and above the soul of the playwright and its own individuality. So, when we review the art of poetry as broadly as we can from the most inward types of lyrical poetry to the most social types of dramatic festival, I think we can see emerging into fuller and fuller light something of the nature of a conflict between the poet's desire to retire wholly into himself and the gradually increasing claims of the human beings with whom he must somehow, as a poet, keep himself in relation. Supposing we were to try to find terms through which to work out the nature of this psychological tension, it seems to me that the most extreme form in which we could legitimately express this tension would be in the antithesis between ' dream ' and ' history.' The dream is the most inward of experiences ; history, if we stress its aspect of accident and contingency, the most outward and objective, and apparently the most independent or defiant of the poet's subjectivity. No doubt the dream has an aspect of being accidental and unwilled, and this shows how merely relative are the terms of the antithesis. Still, I think that if we could envisage the problem of art under the formula, ' To relate the world of dreams to the world of history,' we should be doing the best that the present stage of our dialectic could warrant.

So far we have been carrying on the argument with special reference to the art of literature. But since in accordance with the title of this chapter, I shall have occasion for much employment of the verb, to see, and of the noun, vision : and since I shall be using them, to a large extent at all events in the most simple and literal sense, I should ask the reader to keep in prominence those arts in which the sense of sight and the power of visual imagination play at least the chief rôle—the art of painting, for example. In general, I shall go to that form of art, whatever it be, from which I can most easily, or most exactly, illustrate my argument. The task, however, will always remain of discovering whether the results so obtained are capable of being universalised ; and if they are not, the chances are that the matter has been wrongly stated even for the particular art in question. The challenge must always be brought forward to a judgment supposed to be true of one particular art, say, that of painting : What is stated of this art with its implication of the visible and the visual may here hold good ; but does it follow that it holds good of the other arts, poetry, music, architecture, etc. ?   And if not, why not ?

PLASTICITY AND VISION

(2)

Suppose I look at an object—any object—a tree or a house. I recognise it as real and react to it accordingly. But if I interpose between it and my eyes a series of optical instruments—a telescope, first the narrow end to my eye, then the broad end ; then instruments with coloured lenses ; I shall see the object in all sorts of different ways. Take one of the cases—the wrong end of the telescope. Here I see the object very small and a long way off. In consequence, it provokes a kind of impression that it does not generally arouse. It looks beautiful, perhaps, while before it was only commonplace, an ordinary cottage before, it becomes a cottage in a fairy tale. Quaint associations rush up uncalled. I don't know why they should have come up. They are from ' the unconscious.' Here the term seems very appropriate, and not at all likely to mislead. At the very least, it indicates that power of the imagination through which it comes unwilled.

The cottage has been ' distanced ' by looking through the wrong end of the telescope, and the telescope has become very literally a ' medium.' In a most remarkable piece of writing,[1] one of the most powerful contributions to æsthetic theory that I have read before the days of analytical psychology, Mr. Edward Bullough elucidates and illustrates a principle of ' distance ' offered as a conception sufficiently general to apply to every type of art or even of beauty. ' Distance ' is, of course, used in a metaphorical sense ; Mr. Bullough mentions, indeed, that spatial or literal distance is a particular case of the general psychological concept. I venture to suggest that he does not make quite

[1] *"Psychical Distance " as a Factor in Art and an Æsthetic Principle.* British Journal of Psychology, June, 1912.

enough of this particular case. It seems to me not unimportant to observe that the stars are beautiful because, for one reason among many others, they are very far away. And I wish somewhat to stress my illustration of the wrong end of the telescope as something that affords us a starting point of almost unique advantage ; first, because the telescope turned the wrong way does actually ' distance ' the object in a very literal way ; and second, because the glass lenses of the instrument and their relation to each other, very really and literally constitute a ' medium ' through which the object is seen. Entirely in accordance with the view of the article in question, I should urge that the effect of the inverted telescope is to cut off or inhibit or render unnecessary the normal or economic reactions of life ; while somehow other reactions are brought into play that the undistanced object did not draw out. Now, here is the point where a ' psychology of the unconscious ' might begin to help us to understand what these reactions really are, or what sort of content they imply. We shall not at present do more than suggest, say, that the cottage in the beautiful remote distance of the inverted telescope becomes *malgré nous*—' unconsciously '—a cottage in a fairy world.

Again, consider the awfully unpleasant effect produced by looking at nature through certain combinations of blatantly coloured red and yellow glass, familiar in a certain type of bathroom window, a kind of sick Apocalypse, a combination of jaundice and the last judgment. Nature is ' distanced,' psychologically distanced, by the coloured glass. But the last judgment feeling is not merely an association. We can't help having it.

' A way of viewing nature '—' seeing the object through a medium '—' distanced '—these phrases

88

have each their own meaning. They do not mean
quite the same thing. Nevertheless they indicate a
certain convergence. Looking at nature through
red glass, one cannot help having the feeling of a
lurid last judgment. It is not pleasant, and one
would rather choose another type of glass to look
through. Perhaps one may choose one's glass, but
having chosen and having passed the glass before
one's eyes, the effect is just there. One either makes
the best of it, or rejects it altogether. But now
supposing the 'medium' is a camera, one can,
within certain limits, and by dint of screwing and
pushing, secure a 'distanced' view of nature not
absolutely given, but alterable within certain limits
and, within limits, to one's liking. And here there
is room for a little technique as to the manner
of screwing and pushing.

Again—and this illustration is more important,
because it is the last step we can take without actually
bringing us into the region of art—suppose I look
into a large mirror in which I can see the room reflected. In *Phantastes, a Fairy Romance for Men
and Women*, George Macdonald makes the observation that a commonplace room reflected in a mirror
becomes like a room in a poem. Plato was profoundly wrong when he thought that holding a
mirror up to nature was only a rather brilliant form
of imitation. What he did not see was that all the
right-handed things on the hither side of the mirror
become left-handed things through the looking-glass ;
and you never know your friend's nose is to the side
till you see him reflected in a mirror. Seeing things
in a mirror is, therefore, a quite peculiar and very
instructive form of psychological distance. It may
be a very pleasurable form of æsthetic experience
indeed, though it is not quite art. If you begin to
talk about what you see, you may become an artist :

and George Macdonald wrote a short story, enshrined in *Phantastes,* based upon the psychological
distance afforded by the mirror, that is a complete,
pure and beautiful little work of art.

Now from the mirror to the picture itself is not a
very far cry. They are both of them reflections of
something outside or beyond themselves, or, keeping
to our idiom, they are glimpses or views of things
other than themselves. Here I am bound to
anticipate the criticism that pictures need not be
representative of anything. We shall have to consider in detail, later on, the question whether pictures
are or are not essentially representative. In the
meantime, I am content to accept a childish or naive
conception of pictorial art. For I think that in
æsthetic, childish and naive conceptions are important.

It is, as it were, of set purpose that I am here
employing language of a certain kind of crudity. I
am implying that the picture gives you a means—or
gives the painter a means—of seeing a bit of nature
anew after the analogy of the mirror. Since, however, you see in a mirror only things actually present
outside it—say, a bit of nature ; and since you see
in a picture things not actually present, but that
may have happened long ago, we shall have to add
that what you see may be not only ' a bit of
nature,' but also a ' bit of history.'

And now we are able to state the precise difference
between the mirror reflection and the picture. It
is *in the nature of the medium through* which the
painter *sees* his ' bit of nature ' or ' bit of history.'
In the first case it was a piece of hard, crystalline,
unplastic stuff that you could shatter or destroy at
a blow, but that otherwise is unalterable and gives
an unalterable effect—an effect in its very nature
crystalline, hard, inorganic and unvital. In the

second case, the artist sees his ' bit of nature '
through a medium that is fundamentally plastic—
that his hands must handle and shape in the moment
of his seeing.   Here the concepts of ' plasticity '
and ' vision ' must be brought together and kept
in the closest possible relation.

First, at the close of our discussion on the selective
meditation of the poet, and then again after our
sketch of the nature of the imagination, we had
proposed to distinguish the empty dreamer, the
mere deviser of phantasies from the genuine artist
through the fact that the latter had to have his
' medium '; and at both these stages medium
presented itself to us as most essentially and simply
just the clay of the earth that the primitive dusky
savage would take up to tell you what he was thinking
about or to let you know the phantasies passing in
his mind.   And the more I think of the matter, the
more convinced I am of the truth of this, and of the
artistic importance of the ' medium ' and of the
philosophical importance of its concept.   From the
beginning of days until now there has been a tremendous suggestion of creativeness in the dust of
the earth.   And all the history of art in every epoch,
and all our experience of art anywhere, only goes to
confirm my belief that the Almighty had the correct
idea in His head in the beginning.   The dust of the
earth, moistened—clay, chalk moistened—with water
or oil—marble, bricks, stone—there is a principle
of continuity and evolution here that begins in dust,
but that everywhere ramifies, diverges and presents
new possibilities.   Whether you choose water or oil
to moisten your earth is a point of divergence of
extraordinary significance, indeed, but only typical
of the branch-like divergencies that one finds on
the ' technical ' side of art.

And there must be a primitive sensuousness and

sensuality in the artist towards his medium—or there is nothing at all. It is the ' feel ' of the wet clay, the ' feel ' of the pianoforte keys that counts.

A French writer is said to have remarked that the sight of white paper and a pen gave him feelings of strong emotion akin to that of sexuality. And that, or something like that, must always be the seductive power of the ' medium.' It is necessary to emphasise the ' earthy ' quality of it. It is " earthy, sensual "—and I have no objection to adding the third of St. Paul's trilogy of epithets—" devilish." For there is, and must be, something dæmonic and compulsive in the fascination which his earthy medium exercises upon the artist.

But as well as exercising this dæmonic compulsion upon the artist, *watching* him at his work, *watching* him mould and chisel and carve, must in turn exercise a kind of dæmonic fascination upon people who will never be able themselves to do what he does. The *terribilita* of Michael Angelo at his work is a good illustration—how he " fascinates and is intolerable " as the bits of marble fly in a kind of shining white rainbow from his chisel. That is to say, the people who understand, who really apprehend, in imagination and emotion, the work of a Michael Angelo can never be content merely to look at the finished product. Even though they could not themselves do the smallest bit of real sculpture or painting, they must nevertheless feel what it is like to chisel or paint. And of this appreciation in general, the art of criticism in so far as it is an art, must take full account. This does not make criticism just an indefinitely feeble kind of painting or sculpture. Something will have to be said by and by to justify criticism in its own right. Nevertheless the basal fascination of the medium must be felt by the critic if he is to be a real critic and not some kind of dilettante philosopher or archæologist. It must lie at the root of all he has to say about the art he is trying to evaluate. And this, of course, is to be taken to hold good, in a more general way of the recipient or appreciative spirit as opposed to the creative.

Medium, therefore, is something that links together the artist, his critic and his public, in a very special way. But if so, we should need, should we not, to consider the case of the interpretive actress? By such a logic she becomes quite obviously the ' medium ' of the dramatic poet. And this is unquestionably true in fact. ' Medium ' then can just as well be typified by the players and the dancers in drama as by the clay and the marble elsewhere. What is important here to observe is that the actress is an artist in her own right, or the dancers are artists in their own right. The condition of dramatic art is that poet, actress and dancers somehow meet. They all, somehow express themselves through a common medium. I should not say, therefore, just that the actress or the dancer was the medium.

For she can distinguish between herself as centre and creative source and herself as medium which she uses to express that other self, just as the potter uses the clay as the medium of his self-expression. Clay in the hands of the potter was taken as the most primitive, as the most primeval, type of the medium of art. Alongside this we are now compelled to place the human body as equal in its claim to typify the material medium through which alone art is possible, and through which alone it can become the expression and the satisfaction of a primeval and everlasting human need. And yet because the human body is so used only in its life and its movement, we must attribute vision to the mind which animates and moves it. ' Plasticity and vision,' therefore, must be thought comprehensively enough to include this case. It will be our subsequent task to inquire how far this comprehensiveness is harmonious with significance and precision.

CHAPTER IV

VISION AND CONVENTION

> We receive but what we give
> . . . From the soul itself must issue forth
> A light, a glory, a fair luminous cloud
> Enveloping the Earth.
>
> COLERIDGE.

Have men the faculty of comprehending the universe within their minds, or is the mind indeed a talisman, with which they annihilate the laws of time and space ? Science will oscillate for a long time between these two equally inexplicable mysteries. In any case, however, it is certain that inspiration unfolds to the poet innumerable transfigurations that resemble the magic phantasmagoria of our dreams. A dream is probably the natural outlet of this strange power, when it is unemployed. BALZAC

> . . . Thoughts, that voluntarie move
> Harmonious numbers.
>
> MILTON

(1)

SINCE under the concept, or general formula, ' plasticity and vision,' we mean to include the dramatic poet's ' vision ' of the world through the bodies of the actors who interpret his play, or the dancer's ' vision ' whose medium is her own body, it is clear that the main intention of the formula must be taken as metaphorical or analogical. Yet since there are certain cases where the medium is plastic, in a literal sense, like clay ; and where the vision comes through the eye of sense, as when one has a vision of the heavens through the glass in the windows of Chartres Cathedral, a certain care must be exercised not to allow the accent to fall altogether over upon the merely analogical significance of the formula. A reservation must be made in favour of certain cases where its application seems to have literal truth.

Let us think, for a moment, of the mediæval craftsman, a member of the guild of stained glass workers, who has to adorn the new cathedral with a window representing the Madonna. Is it too imaginative, I wonder, to conceive that he asks himself, " Where shall I look for the Madonna to know what she is like— the *Mater Coelestis?* " Is it too imaginative to suppose that he looks up into the sky in the hope of seeing her there ? I scarcely think so ; and at all events it is certain that many people *have* looked at the visible heavens in the attempt to discover her there. Suppose, then, the mediæval glass-worker looks up into the sky in this intention. He cannot find her. His orientation to the sky is too commonplace, too intellectual, too merely practical.

Like all the generations of at least northern European mankind, he has to look at the clouds every day before he goes to his work to see if it is going to rain ; and his habitual pre-occupation about rain makes his attitude to the heavens far too utilitarian ; and so he cannot see the *Mater Coelestis*.

So he devises this device. He goes into the cathedral—newly finished, except for the glazing of the windows—and between the sky and himself he inserts blue glass, coloured like the sky, and behold, the *Mater Coelestis* appears, and at last he knows what she is like.

The image of the Madonna that the mediæval workman projects upon the sky through the magical efficacy of his medium comes from himself. The *Mater Coelestis* seems to be in the heavens, but, in fact he finds her there only because she was first within himself. He receives only what he has given.

When the old workman looks at the sky with the eyes of every day common sense, he cannot see the

Mater Coelestis, but he can see the rain clouds, he can gauge the direction of the wind, and he can tell whether or not there is likely soon to be a storm. Even there it is true to say, in another sense, that he receives but what he gives ; and that it is only in virtue of past experience that he can so discern the signs of the times. The two ways of looking at the sky do nevertheless show entirely different aims or intentions. They typify two distinct attitudes towards the heavens, or two distinct orientations to life. We may call the one the artistic, and the other the practical. Now though art is sometimes practical, and though in the commonplace attitude towards nature that our everyday life demands, perceptions of beauty often blend with our dull and practical life, the two orientations are nevertheless well differentiated, and clearly distinguishable from each other.

In both orientations, it may be admitted, we receive only what we have already given. Yet the manner of our giving and receiving is, in each case, so different, that we must be at pains to show wherein the essential difference lies.

How do we perceive objects as they are for intellectual knowledge ? How do we see objects in such wise that we think or feel them to be beautiful ?

The first of these two questions has been the main pre-occupation of Western philosophy almost from its very beginning. Almost from the time when, in Greece, philosophy became articulate as such, its chief problem has been to understand how it is possible to ' know ' an object. So urgent has this problem always been for the Western mind, that it has pursued it to the exclusion of other, perhaps equally legitimate, problems of philosophy ; and in consequence of this exclusive bias, it has never been able even to formulate its problem correctly. When at last the deeper psychological insight of our own age is urging upon

97

philosophy that it cannot state, let alone solve, its problem of knowledge, until due recognition has been made that there are other problems, perhaps equally urgent, the moment seems ripe for an attempt to formulate some of these. In especial, it is legitimate to ask, and it is here our immediate task to formulate, the second of our two questions : How do we see objects in such wise that we think or feel them to be beautiful ?

Even in the perception of an object that is directed towards knowledge, it is clear that the object does not merely thrust itself on the mind, but that it acquires significance through what the mind itself has to bestow upon the object. Even in knowledge, it is true that something must be given by the mind before anything can be received. Perception takes place through the continual presence or emergence of images more or less unobserved that in Bergson's language, "insert" themselves in the nascent perception, coalesce with it, and in this insertion and coalescence constitute the very perception itself. Not to go further afield than his little book on dreams, we may take Bergson's apt and beautiful illustrations of the way in which the mind ' perceives ' things that are not really in the object perceived, as sufficiently convincing on this point.[1] The more easily the perceptual process takes place, the less chance there is of the emergence of the images, as images, into consciousness. It is only when there is a certain difficulty, a certain lack of smoothness and habitual efficiency in the process, that images may render themselves up to our observation.

Thus even in knowledge of outer objects through perception, the most accurate perception can come about only in virtue of an image content that is supplied from within. " Perception is never a mere

[1] *Dreams*. Eng. translation, pp. 41ff.

contact of the mind with the object present ; it is impregnated with memory images, which complete it, as they interpret it."[1]

Suppose, however, that not knowledge, but the pleasures of the imagination, are in question. Let the imagination be free to wander as it will. Left to itself, it is too free ; and so it seeks to express itself, or to fill out its too formless or colourless images, with the clear forms and the bright colours of the outer sensuous world. Within the tide of the imagination, then, there may arise something that looks like perception. This kind of perception, however, is the inverse of ' real ' perception, or it proceeds by an inverse method. We may define the perceptual process as it is for knowledge through Bergson's formula of the insertion of images within the nucleus of sensation. The sensation or the nascent perception constitutes a point of stability. It is the pivot around which the whole process turns.

When the imagination is in the ascendency, we can no longer speak of images as inserted within even the *soi-disant* perception. It is rather as if the sensations were taken up and inserted within the continuum of the imagination. The imagination governs ; and the sensuous is of avail only when the sensation is suitable for the image. In the first case the image was of avail only when it was suitable for the perception. In the second case, the imagination is the determining factor. In the words of a French writer, the imaginative mind " inserts the material into the spiritual."

At first sight it may seem as if thus to oppose ' knowledge ' to ' imagination ' were begging the whole question, since by our very pre-supposition we do not know what knowledge is. I am concerned, however, not with a theory of knowledge, but only

[1] Bergson. *Matter and Memory*. Eng. translation. Chap. IV., p. 170.

with the relative distinction between knowledge as required for the practical management of affairs, and imagination as an obviously unsuitable guide in practical life, and defined through the negation of practical value.

True, once again, the practical mind requires imagination before it can be practically effective ; and the imaginative artist may require all the practical powers of the engineer before he can be creative in art. The two orientations are nevertheless distinct, and well differentiated from each other. In this sense, then, the relative distinction between knowledge and imagination is as clear as any distinction can be within the differentiated powers of the human mind.

One remark, however, is worth making in this context. It is possible that there may be whole fields of the imaginative life where sensation does not enter, or does not enter as an essential factor ; just as there may be whole fields of possibly non-imaginative experience like thought, where sensation does not, or need not, enter, but where imagery seems to be an essential, though subordinate, factor. Those realms of the imagination, however, where sensation plays no essential part, do not belong to art ; and so again, we are not now concerned with them.

Can we catch the artist in the moment of transition between his mere perception of an object of ordinary intellectual or utilitarian interest and the dawning of a new interest in the object in virtue of which he feels he would like to paint it or write a poem about it ? I think we can. Even the least artistic of us have had the experience that some object—persistently dull and commonplace—suddenly becomes clothed in a new and mysterious light, and we feel that even we, if we had the poet's technique or the rudiments of the painter's gift, could see visions and dream dreams.

It is at this point that we must pass from the

poverty of our own minds to the richness of the mind of the artist. He can do what we cannot do. He can bring up between himself and the object that medium of his vision that he thinks will most intensify it in its imaginative character and that will most completely make it vision indeed. This bringing up of the medium, we might almost regard as the authoritative gesture, as the act of pyschological command, that exorcises the sterile spirit of the practical intellect and liberates the creative forces of the imagination.

Alike in perception and in the imaginative process where the sensuous is thus invoked to fill out the content of the imagination, the co-ordination of more than one sensory organ may be involved. Sight and touch, for example, are continually supplementing and limiting each other in ordinary perception ; and the same is true in the artist's handling of his medium in all the graphic and plastic arts. It is probable, however, that the artistic process involves a much higher degree of reciprocity between the tactile and the visual than perception ever does.[1]

In thus comparing the two processes, and since in each the mind seems to give its own contribution of images, would it not be possible to say that in both cases these images came " out of the unconscious ? " When it is said that in the act of vision secured through the plasticity of the medium, images " come out of the unconscious " and enter into the totality of the vision, may it not just as well be said that in perception the images to be inserted in the perception come from exactly the same source, viz., the unconscious ? In so far as, in both cases, there are images, it will indeed be right to trace them to the same source. The essential difference, however, lies in the practical

---

[1] For an account of the co-ordination of the tactile and the visual, cf. *Mind and Medium in Art*, p. 38. E. Bullough. British Journal of Psychology, Vol. XI., Part 1.

character of perception. In so far as images arise within the perceptual process and fail to blend or to coalesce with the perception, but become detached from it, these images are useless and irrelevant. Perception, therefore, does not offer scope for images that begin to assume any kind of separate or individual existence. Imagery, as such, tends to destroy perception, and floods of imagery will change the entire process and take it altogether away from the perceptual. When, on the other hand, images rush in upon the mind of the artist as he watches the object transforming itself through his medium, these images are precious. They are the very content of his vision, or at least they may become such. The richer the flow of imagery, the greater at all events are the resources at his command. The content of the unconscious is welcomed. In this sense, then, art involves, and must involve, " the unconscious " in a way that perception for knowledge never can involve it, and must not admit it.

(2)

As in Chapter II on the Nature and Origin of the Imagination, I proposed the view that image in the more restricted sense of memory image or phantasy image is not altogether different from dream, or that dream and imagery represent perhaps an altogether continuous order of mental phenomena ; so now I return to consideration of the dream from the point of view at once of this chapter and of the continuity which I have supposed in the former.

When language was used that seemed to imply that an image ' wanted ' to express itself, or that there were images in the minds of all of us ' seeking ' some kind of external expression or embodiment, we

should have to ask : Wherefore this urge ? Why do
some images seem so ardently to ' want ' this
expression ? or, from the other point of view, why are
some objects so suitable for calling forth images out of
the unconscious, while other objects stimulate no
interest and create no imagery ? The answer would be,
in keeping with the general principles of analytical
psychology, that we must look for this urge, that we
must explain this disquietude, in something much
larger than the minuscule of an image. The image,
that is to say, might be regarded as a tiny outcrop of a
vast psychical mine lying further below the surface.

Are the phenomena of dreaming, then, continuous
with those of images ?

Every evidence goes to show that dreams, as a
whole, seem to ' want ' to express themselves in some
way. When a man forgets his dreams or ignores them,
the dreams go on dreaming themselves over and over
again even in sleep ; but they also, in virtue of being
ignored, try to dream themselves *through objects*.
The tendency to dream, that is to say, remains
operative in the daytime, so that a man cannot
smoothly adapt himself to his environment in the
accepted manner of the present, or in the fashion
required by the latest civilisation. It is as if the
archaic which, as we have seen, expresses itself *par
excellence* in dreams, represented an orientation unacceptable to the people with whom he has to deal
and with whom he has to find rapport. He tends to
the dream attitude even when awake. Dreams may
be oppressive by night, but the dream attitude by day
will cause its own obscure and indefinite suffering,
will beget its own inexplicable confusion. Swinburne
has seen the truth of this principle, and has employed
it with an exquisite felicity in the *Atalanta*. After
the opening chorus, the song of spring in honour of the
gods, Althæa enunciates the counter subject, that of

the uncomprehended doom against which even prayer
is of no avail :—

> I marvel what men do with prayers awake
> Who dream and die with dreaming . . .
> For if sleep have no mercy, and man's dreams
> Bite to the blood and burn into the bone,
> What shall this man do waking ?

So long as man's dreams are a divine mystery, they
are also an inevitable destiny. Nothing could illustrate this better than the tragic issue of the recent
Everest expedition. The cinematograph film as
exhibited in London is the most convincing proof of
the ' unconsciousness ' of the ' Natural Science ' of
England. Confronted with the religious attitude of
India and Thibet, the unrecognised within the minds
of the explorers was profoundly stirred ; but as
unrecognised was projected upon Mount Everest
itself, which became invested with divine terrors.
The film showed us " a fight with nature." But so
long as man fights with nature, nature will always win.
The Thibetan lamas rightly prophesied failure. Yet
surely Everest should be ascended. May one pay
one's tribute to the forerunners in the hope that the
ascension will eventually be made in a profounder
comprehension of Nature and of the East ?

The dream, then, as mysterious, unintelligible,
ignored, will find some uncontrolled and inappropriate
expression. This unrecognised expression of the dream
may be described as dreaming through objects.
It will, of course, show all degrees of unrecognition
and unconsciousness. When objects are invested
with blind terrors, and nature becomes a series of
magical phantasmagoria, it may indicate a very
profound unconsciousness ; and the man thus dreaming through objects, save that he has his eyes open,
may differ but little from the dreamer in sleep. As
a rule, however, certain objects inspire the dream-like
state more easily than others ; and when a man

becomes interested in the magical spell which a particular object exerts upon him, his interest implies recognition of the sources of the magic, and may enable him to turn the fascination into channels that subserve an intention which is his own.

In this way, dreams on a larger scale become extraordinarily like the images on a smaller scale, that, as Bergson says, " impregnate " the perception of real objects. " Dreaming through objects " might, therefore, become an essential phase in the totality of an experience of intrinsic value ; just as the " insertion " of the image in a perception, or the " impregnation " of it with the image is an essential condition of perpetual knowledge.

Here is an example.

A certain philosopher had been dreaming, by night, about caves, but had not paid much heed to his dreams. One day, in his meditative rambles about the countryside, he came to a cave ; its mystery intrigued him, and he was enticed to enter. It happened to be the late afternoon sunshine, and the level rays of the sun were finding their way past him along the floor of the cave. They made unwonted and delightful shadows, and the shape of his own body was thrown distortedly upon the rock-wall. He enjoyed himself very much in his own way—pleased with the unusual lights and shadows, and nobly entertained with his own reflections about them. He waited for some time to enjoy the seductive tranquillity of the place, until sunset cut short his opportunity ; and then he went home and wrote the seventh book of *The Republic*.

What was he doing all the time, if not dreaming about the rebirth of the soul ? Had he been sound asleep he would have been dreaming about caves all the same—the descent of the deliverer and the resurrection of the liberated ; but in this waking dream of his, he had at once a real cave to help him out with it, and a real philosophic purpose to make him conscious of it, however partial and imperfect his consciousness.

This process of dreaming through objects may just as accurately be formulated as the projection of an unconscious content upon an object. The cave ' in the unconscious,' the symbol, perhaps, of the womb into which one must enter before one can be reborn into the sunlight of the intelligible world, is ' projected ' on to the cave—I had almost said—' in the real world,' save that my terminology would not be quite harmonious with Plato's. But I can say, with safety, ' projected on to the cave in the world of rocks and hills and ocean, of visible shadows and sunlight.'

We have emerged, then, at a point of view from which there appears to be no difference in principle between the insertion of an image in the quasi-perceptual process through which the artist views his object through his medium and this projection of the larger ' unconscious ' content of the dream. Indeed, as the artist handles his medium, we should now need to assert with less reservation that by so doing he is ' dreaming through the object.' We should only need to observe in addition that, in the actual work of artistic construction, such dreaming through the object will be a slow and complex process. Within this larger and more laborious whole, we shall be able to detect, as its *modus operandi,* the continual insertion of smaller images upon the object as seen through the medium.[1]

Supposing, then, there be a real continuity between image and dream, let us return to Mr. Bullough's principle of psychological distance. It will become apparent that ' distancing ' is closely related to

[1] Cf. the " *images motrices* " and " *images de traduction* " of Arreat. *Vide Mind and Medium in Art,* p. 37.   British Journal of Psychology, XI., 1.

projection. Distance in Mr. Bullough's view is effected
by cutting off the normal or economic reactions of
life, and so allowing a new reaction or a new system
of reactions to take their place. I think we may
express entire agreement with this. It is the nature
of the new system of reactions that we should wish
to explore in the light of what has since been discovered about 'the unconscious.' The idea of
projection gives us a very much more positive cue to
the nature of the reaction that supervenes upon the
recession of the practical demands of the world. As
distanced, the object becomes endowed with 'unconscious' contents ; and in so far as analytical psychology appears to be such a powerful means of
discovering their nature and origin, it should certainly
place us more securely on the path towards a better
understanding of the nature of art, or, at least, of the
processes of art.

Projection, then, is correlated to distance. It is
important to emphasise this, because it is only on a
more or less distant object that one can 'throw out'
things. Possibility of the projection of unconscious
contents involves the separation of the thrower from
the object upon which he throws. It is an aspect of
separation ; and this aspect has, it seems to me, been
splendidly elucidated by Mr. Bullough.

(3)

But there is something else implied in projection,
which is not brought out or which is not fully brought
out through the principle of distance alone. Schopenhauer[1] suggests that in experience of beauty the
perceiving subject does not stand over against the
beautiful object in the same way that the knowing

[1] *The World as Will and Idea.* Book III.

subject is opposed to the object of knowledge.
Perhaps even it is not quite appropriate to speak of
subject and object in beauty. There has, at least,
been a vague tradition to that effect, never perhaps
achieving philosophical precision of expression until
Schopenhauer. The parallel tradition in the case of
mysticism has had a much more powerful and vigorous
expression ; and in this respect it may be not un-
instructive to attempt to link up the mystical
experience with that of beauty. Be that as it may,
mysticism must not at present be allowed to involve
us in its alluring and seductive marvels. What is
important is that in Schopenhauer we do find a very
vigorous and clear re-casting of the old nebulous
tradition in regard to beauty. He asserts that in
æsthetic contemplation the terms of the antithesis,
perceiving subject and object perceived, do not exist
for the experience of beauty in the way that they
exist for knowledge and the knowledge-experience.
His whole contention is elaborated with illustration
from the beauty of art and of nature at once of a
fitness and magnificence that makes the third book
of *The World as Will and Idea* such a landmark both
in the history of æsthetic and of philosophy in general.
In view, therefore, of a tradition that is at least as old
as Plato, if not much older, and of such a striking
crystallisation of that tradition in Schopenhauer, I
hesitate to accept Mr. Bullough's principle of psychological distance as anything like a *complete* account
of the matter. I do think that his principle takes us
a very long way, and I cannot sufficiently express my
admiration of the way in which it is worked out and
illustrated. I also note that he speaks of " the antimony of distance."[1] That is to say, there must be a
definite limit to the psychological distance at which

[1] *Psychical Distance as an Æsthetic Principle.* British Journal of
Psychology, V. 2, pp. 92 ff.

the object is placed, the law deducible from the work of the great artists being that the distance is the least possible consistent with the effective operation of the principle. The theatre, for example, cannot represent the actions and speech of men and women with a complete realism. It must, however, give as much realism as is possible ; but if it give too much, it would cease to appeal to the artistic emotion of the audience and would speak directly to their human and personal emotions. Heine tells a story of a production of the *Merchant of Venice* in which the sympathies of a woman in the audience were so completely enlisted in favour of Shylock that during the trial scene, she exclaimed, " The poor man is wronged ! " She failed sufficiently to distance the character of the Jew and so her relation to it became personal and non-dramatic.

This " antimony of distance," I should agree, takes us a long way and shows us a great deal. And yet, I feel also, in the last resort, that there is something in the concept of distance which leaves altogether untouched that aspect of the experience of beauty upon which Schopenhauer so strongly insists—the union, or the apparent union, of the perceiving subject with the object, that may in certain cases almost nullify the subject-object antithesis in experience of beauty that is typical or profound

If we develop the implications of projection, if we admit that an ' unconscious content ' is, in the act of seeing in virtue of the plasticity of the medium, projected as the artist directs his vision upon the object, we have also to admit that the object seen must be capable of, as it were, receiving the projection. Not every object is equally suitable for projection. Not every bit of landscape is equally calculated to inspire the landscape painter to the really beautiful landscape painting. There is a suitability, then, in the object. Now I can fancy that at this point I shall be asked if I really mean that some objects are suitable for ' representation ' in painting and some not. I should reply, I think, that so far as the history of art goes, there are objects that no artist has yet found suitable ' to represent.' What I really mean, however, is, that there are many ' bits of nature ' and many ' bits of history ' that have so far thrown out a defiant and successful challenge to every artist and to every type of art: The war, for instance, as a whole, and innumerable ' bits ' of it, still remain unamenable to art. What I should not say is that such things as the war will eventually and completely resist artistic treatment, or for ever fail to inspire the artist. On the other hand, the challenges of these things are not likely to be met effectually except through the creation of new forms of art, and the discovery of new media—the cinema, for instance. I, therefore, once more take up my concept of suitability in the object with its correlative concept of selection and power of selection in the artist. Ruskin's formula that the lover can sing about his lost love, but the miser cannot sing about his lost gold, is a useful one at this stage of the argument.

How, then, can an object—a ' bit of history,' or ' a bit of nature,' in Zola's phrase, *un coin de la nature*—be made suitable to receive the projection of the unconscious ? We should at first try to answer this question merely through illustration, analogy or metaphor ; and to be content with such treatment of the subject during the remainder of this chapter, leaving over to a following chapter the extremely difficult task of translating our analogies into terms of adequate psychological precision.

Just as the artist has the power of psychological distance, and in ' distancing ' also projects, he has also the correlative power of bringing the object closer to himself. The analogue of the process would be given if, in some space of unknown or unnameable dimensional quality, one could look through both ends of the telescope at once. In the real artistic process, however, of mediating himself to the object by clay or marble or paint, this is what the artist achieves. This is what it is the very nature of the artistic process to accomplish. As through projection, the object is given something that it did not possess, so also something is taken away from the object that otherwise, or in a non-artistic view of it, had evidently belonged to it.

What is it that is taken away from the object, or *how* does the artist see the object as deprived of something that is otherwise known to belong to it ?

(4)

Theories of *Einfühlung* have been frequently illustrated through the idea of life or of something vital and life-like that is 'felt to' an object otherwise, or in another relation, recognised to be lifeless. The water reflecting the sunlight is not really living, yet Aeschylus speaks of its "innumerable laughter"; and only living things can laugh. There must, however, be an opposite or obverse of *Einfühlung*, in which a living object is felt as dead, or in which some kind of lifelessness is felt as belonging to it.[1] This obverse process is well illustrated where the convention of art demands that an object full of the irregularity and illogical spontaneity of life must be seen as formalised, rhythmicised or reduced to some kind of regularity and order. Architecture or that phase of the art in which vital, organic forms

[1] Cf. especially *Abstraktion und Einfühlung*. Wilhelm Worringer, München.

like the lily or the vine or the acanthus are conventionalised through the geometrical necessities of decoration, seems to me to illustrate this principle with a peculiar simplicity. It is necessary to deprive these plant forms of their vital irregularity before they can fall into focus within the impression of the architectural whole.

This principle, so obvious in architecture, can be traced in the continuity of its operation through every form of art in which any kind of living thing is represented. Before the living thing can be seen artistically through the given medium, it must in some degree be deprived of its vitality.

It would thus appear that everywhere—in the forms of art we have been discussing—there is on one side an attribution of life to the object—an unconscious attribution—in the very moment when, on some other side, the object is deprived of its life. The rocks and the glacier—known to be inorganic and lifeless—become, for the artist as he paints them, the haunt of dragons ; but the living trees and grass that clothe the rocks are rhythmicised and ordered according to the formal quality that must be felt in every picture.

Now the line of thought upon which we wish to enter is that the more the medium is of such a nature as to lead the artist's vision outward to the object, the more he tends to endow with life the object that he sees or thinks he sees ; and the more the medium is of such a nature as to darken or blur or obscure the artist's vision of the object, the more he tends to deprive the object of its life. In other words the representative movement or orientation in art tends to vitalise the inorganic, while the formal or rhythmical movement or orientation tends to devitalise the organic. In still other words, the more the artist's interest is absorbed in an external object

the more he ' sees ' it living or endows it with life ;
while if the outer object only serve as a means of
initiating his interest which, in its development,
flows back more and more to his own mind or soul,
the less life he sees in the object, the more he deprives
it of its vital qualities.

Could we not here bring in once more the idea of
projection, and generalise it ; so that instead of
saying that the artist deprives the object of its life,
we should say that he projects death on to the living
object ? I think we shall find that we cannot
effectively generalise the idea of projection in this
way. For projection implies distance ; and the
moment or phase in experience of beauty with which
we are now concerned is not satisfactorily explained
through the idea of distance. That aspect of the
object through which it is felt to be one with the
subject, or through which the subject is felt to be
living in the object can only be understood through
the opposite of distance. Projection, however,
emphasises the *distance* of the object from the perceiving subject. There must be an inverse process
or movement which emphasises the *closeness* of the
object to, or even its union with, the subject, in so
far as his experience is of beauty.

Or in other words, the object is no longer felt just
as out there, or over against the subject. Its mere
brute contingency is taken away, or mitigated. The
brute character—which is, of course, also the vital
character—is no longer felt, or is felt less keenly.
The object has been, to however slight an extent,
appropriated by, or made one with, the subject ; or
if you like, the subject has gone out to meet, or has
entered into, the object. And we must leave room,
in any æsthetic, for the formulation of this stage in
the experience of beauty where the antithesis of
subject to object. becomes unreal and fades away.

In any complete account of the experience, or taking it in its totality, we do, no doubt, need to state the subject-object relationship. We need to take account of experience of beauty in its genesis and evolution as well as in what it is typically or at its most intense ; and we have admitted, as our initial approach, that orientation of the artist in which he stands *vis-à-vis* the object. As we shall see, however, the enjoyment of music can only be thought with much greater difficulty as the experience of an object. It is far more easily conceived as an experiencing in which any object experienced is, or tends to be, at a vanishing point. And what we find so deeply to characterise music, we shall find, at all events, to be reflected in every form of art.

The movement or moment, of the experience, then, with which we have now to deal is a movement towards the object or of union with the object. Or, approaching the matter from the side of the subject, the movement would be equivalent to a lost or lessening consciousness of the self. This follows as a matter of course. For if the object is a vanishing factor in the experience, so must be the subject. Now, of course, it is obvious that this movement, too, no less than the correlative movement of projection, may be unrecognised by the subject. His loss of himself, his feeling himself one with what before he was only perceiving but now actually seems to be, is taken for granted as the reality. If that is so, or if there be this quality present, however dimly or vaguely, in the experience, it is clear that the accidental character of the object, its mere obtrusion, is either removed or lessened.

The object which rivets the attention of the artist, the *coin de la nature* upon which his gaze is fixed, is initially presented to him in an unsuitable irregularity. The *coin de la nature* cannot just be copied by the landscape painter, nor can the 'bit of history' just be related by the poet. It is somehow made regular. The accidental character is removed from it as a whole, and the accidents of its parts are regularised and made into the accents of a rhythm. It is believed, it is felt, or rather it is just taken for granted, that the accidents and irregularities have become subject to the control of the perceiving creative mind and are in reality no longer accidents but accents, no longer irregularities but rhythm.

Let us take an example. When Dionysus married Ariadne, according to the myth, he placed the wedding crown which he gave her, in the heavens and it shone for ever among the stars. It is clear at once that the sky itself by night is a magnificent object upon which to project this myth, this 'unconscious content.' If you try to do it directly, you are bewildered by the multitude of stars and you cannot disentangle Ariadne's crown from the rest. But when Titian looks at the sky through oil paint, he thinks he can control the heavens ; he thinks he can take away all the stars except eight, and he thinks he can arrange these eight in a crown-like device. The number and order of the stars have become in subjection to him, and it is because he never questions this subjection of the stars to his will, but just takes it for granted, that this movement of his creative power is genuinely 'unconscious' in the same sense as his initial projection of the myth upon the sky was unconscious. This time what he has done is 'unconsciously' to take away the actual accidental irregularities of the stars, as before he had 'unconsciously' bestowed upon them something that in their own right they did not possess. The beautiful, rhythmic ordering of the stars in paint is his way not so much of making believe that he can number and order them as simply of taking for granted that he does so. To project Ariadne's crown upon the stars is at the same time to take away the contingency of their own motion through the heavens. If he does not know where the crown has come from, neither does he render himself aware of the real, eternal, unchangeable orbits of the stars.

This last illustration shows us that it is not necessarily or exclusively the *life* of the object of which it has to be deprived. It is the utter aloofness of the object, its mere reality and occurrence in and for itself which must be taken away from it. Yet one of the things that is, from the point of view of the subject, most accidental, most irregular, most aloof, least capable of assimilation and least under control, is the life of a living object—plant, animal, or man. This is the absolutest thing, the most entirely on its own, the most hopelessly free from possibility of subjection. The way, therefore, in which the artist must see the living creature is by somehow depriving it of that terrible, unamenable, independent power of being alive. Perhaps the finest typification of this in the whole range of art is that affected in sculpture. Typically the object of the sculptor's eye is the naked, warm, living body of man or woman. Typically the medium of the sculptor is stone in its most purely crystalline, cold, colourless, and inorganic aspect—marble. So seeing his object—through marble—the sculptor is able in the highest possible degree to induce the illusion of control over the living thing itself on the side of its absolutest, completest vitality. That is why sculpture is so peculiarly useful as a means of illustrating and of rendering clear to ourselves the conventionalising, regularising, rhythmicising quality or power of art. At no point is the representative tendency of art so complete on every side as in sculpture ; and yet nowhere is the merely imitative function of art so specifically negated. Nowhere as in sculpture is the beauty of the material medium so immediately exhibited to sense. Here the inherent convention found somewhere in all art lies plainly on the surface. Another illustration of this process or moment in the artistic experience is, I think, necessary before we can pass on. It is that of a certain aspect of the spirit of tragedy. Supposing we call, this time, the ' bit of nature or history ' which is before the vision of the tragic dramatist, ' the suffering of the world.' It is upon this suffering that he is to project his myth. But the sheer, brute, contingent and uncontrolled suffering of history will not bear *any* projection of his just as it stands. He must deprive it somehow of its sheerness. Somehow, then, he does manage to take for granted that ' the suffering of the world ' is under *some* control, some human-divine control, the artist's own control, really. That is what the great tragic artists do manage to take for granted and to get taken for granted. It is the terrible, living *aloofness* that they manage to take away from suffering, seeing it as they do through the enigmatic, dark glass of their medium. This gives them the illusion of their control : and in that apparent, rhythmic control, with every artifice of divided and ordered chorus, with every device of measured sound and pattern of related colour, they sing :—

ἰὼ γενεαὶ βροτῶν,
ὡς ὑμᾶς ἴσα καὶ τὸ μηδὲν ζώσας ἐναριθμῶ.
τίς γάρ, τίς ἀνὴρ πλέον
τᾶς εὐδαιμονίας φέρει
ἢ τοσοῦτον ὅσον δοκεῖν
καὶ δόξαντ' 'αποκλῖναι ;
τὸν σόν τοι παράδειγμ' ἔχων,
τὸν σὸν δάιμονα, τὸν σόν, ὦ τλᾶμον Οἰδιπόδα,
βροτῶν
οὐδὲν μακαρίζω . . . . . . [1]

[1] O ye children of men, I count you but as though ye had not been. For what man is there who achieveth aught of happiness save only in the semblance thereof, and in the very semblance, declineth ? With such as thou before mine eyes, and thy destiny, none, dread Œdipus, of mortal men do I call blest . . .

SOPHOCLES, *Œdipus Rex*, 1155 ff.

Ruskin has given a very fine emotional rendering of this conventionalising aspect of the tragic spirit. It is emotional, because ostensibly he does not identify himself with the artistic spirit at all. He is supposed to be speaking from the standpoint of practical truth and of moral values. And yet because from another point of view he recognises the claims of the artistic spirit, if he is not at heart identified with it, his account of the four great representatives of the tragic spirit, Homer, Dante, Shakespeare and Milton, becomes of extraordinary significance and value. Of course, it must be divested of its emotion. Or rather, the unrecognised duality of his standpoint must be made clear and allowed for ; and then the value of the emotion itself will become apparent.

With Dante chiefly in mind, he speaks with a kind of rapt mockery of the poets who " dare to play with the most precious truth (or the most deadly untruths), by which the whole human race listening to them could be informed or deceived." But this is just what the great tragic poets have done. They have thought of truth only as matter for " play," and subject to the conventions and rhythms of play, " all the world their audiences for ever, with pleased ear and passionate heart—and yet to this submissive infinitude of souls, and evermore succeeding and succeeding multitude, hungry for bread of life, they do but play upon sweetly modulated pipes ; with pompous nomenclature adorn the councils of hell ; touch a troubadour's guitar to the courses of the suns ; and fill the openings of eternity, before which prophets have veiled their faces, and which angels desire to look into, with idle puppets of their scholastic imagination . . ."

" Touch a troubadour's guitar to the courses of the suns . . ." That " touch a troubadour's guitar " of Ruskin has always seemed to me the finest and the completest thing that has ever been said about the spirit of tragedy. No doubt, we need to unfold its implications, but I do not think that anyone ever made a profounder suggestion.

This, at all events, is how I should envisage the problem of the conventional, formal, or rhythmic quality of art. But in order to make the attempt towards a closer scrutiny of the artist's psychology in this relation, we must now pass to the consideration of those arts, like music and architecture, where the formal or rhythmic aspect seems to be dominant in contrast with sculpture or painting where, though always present, it seems to be half-concealed in their representative power and to emerge only, as it were, by a kind of implication.

CHAPTER V

The Transition to Music

(1)

THE argument of the previous chapters has been
carried on almost entirely through the concepts of
' vision,' ' seeing,' and the power of the visual, and
with reference to those arts in which the sense of sight
is either of central importance or plays a very large
part.   There is another sense organ, however, through
which, as well as with the eye, the world makes the
greater part of its æsthetic appeal.   The transition
from the eye to the ear is perhaps one of the ways that
help us to envisage the difficult problem of this chapter.
At all events, with the simple question : What about
the ear ? there inevitably follows a demand for
special consideration of the art of music.

It is natural to speak about seeing an object ; but it
is not so natural to speak of ' hearing an object,' and
the absence of naturalness should, I think, be taken
to imply a real difficulty.   True, we do speak of
' hearing a sound,' and a sound is an object.   But I
call attention to the fact that we do not instinctively
speak of ' hearing an object.'   For the purposes of
our argument, that is to say, we have thought the
artistic process in so far as the graphic and plastic arts
were concenrned—and to a large extent dramatic art—
through the formula of ' seeing an object through a

medium.' If the formula were to have the validity
and universality of which we are in search, we ought
to be able to think, say, the art of music, through the
corresponding formula, ' hearing an object through a
medium,' and in this, I suggest, we should have a
radical distortion of psychological reality.

Let us refer once more to architecture or to the arts
of quasi-geometrical design—the decoration of the
cathedral floor, or the purely decorative use of mosaic
in so far as it is confined to pattern making, and
appears to represent nothing. These are arts of the
visual—or arts in which the sense of sight is the
dominant one—and yet we encounter the same feeling
of distortion when we try to think them as ' seeing a
bit of nature ' through a medium.

These considerations will perhaps go to reinforce the
doubts raised in the preceding chapter as to whether
our initial view of the artist as directing his gaze
outwardly upon nature would take us all the way
through the realm of art.

There has been a tradition in the history of æsthetic
theory which has attempted to group together on the
one hand the arts of sculpture, painting, and possibly
that of literature, and to oppose them to the arts of
music, architecture, and quasi-geometrical design on
the other ; and to call the former group representative
and the latter non-representative. The naïve view,
at all events, is that a poem tells you *about* something
that happened, or that a picture represents something
that exists or might exist in the natural world ; whereas
a building does not, and cannot, either relate a story
about something, or represent anything beyond itself.
My contention is that this naïve view is not merely
naïve, but will issue, if we follow it carefully, in
something that is of real philosophical import.

And that is why I have invited the reader to accept
as an initial point of view, the emphasis laid upon the

artist's outward orientation—his turning towards outward nature as the apparent source of his vision.

Much has been said in modern critical and æsthetic literature that goes to cast scorn upon the naïve view, or at the least, to cast doubt upon the value of the distinction between art that apparently represents, and art that evidently does not. There is, in especial, a movement in present day criticism that emphasises the formal or rhythmic qualities of painting—a kind of art which, if art is ever anywhere ' representative,' is surely not to be denied the typical qualities of representation.

I recognise too much that is of value in the contemporary movement to regard its standpoint with disrespect. This need not hinder me from demanding a full analysis of the antithesis between the representative and the non-representative arts. If it is only a superficial distinction, an analysis should lead us to discard it. If it is not superficial, it is incumbent upon us to discover its psychological ground. Whether the distinction in question, then, prove to be only apparent or on the surface, or whether it turn out to be profound, the *prima facie* challenge which it certainly makes cannot in any case be ignored.

There is a difference, however, between the point of view that discovers a moment of representation, and a moment of rhythm or form in all art and the point of view which envisages a classification of the arts as representative, on the one hand, and non-representative on the other. The view to which I should eventually wish to lead up, is that the discovery of the moment of representation and of the moment of rhythm in all art, can be deepened into, and will eventually compel us to accept, the principle that an art differentiates itself as a natural species either through emphasis upon the representative and the subordination of the formal, or by the development of its formal power over and above its representative and the due subordination of the latter to the former. Here again, however, it is a question of tendency, and not of absoluteness. We have to keep in view, moreover, the problems involved in the synthesis of such a severely rhythmic art as that of music with so energetically representative an art as that of the dramatic. Is music-drama most typically an art of rhythm or an art of representation ? Answer to this question must be held over ; but if we ask it now, it will help to define the spirit in which we must proceed with our argument.

Assuredly the formal, conventional or non-representative character of the most realistic of the arts is never absent. But it has, in most cases, been found a matter of which it is extraordinarily hard to give a convincing account. If, therefore, there were any chance of apprehending its nature a little more easily in those cases where it is—or appears to be—dominant, as in pure music or architecture, it should be possible to return to the more apparently representative types of art, and to unearth their qualities of form and rhythm, concealed because of their representative value, but none the less pervasive and essential.

The same critical denial of real force in the antithesis, representative *versus* non-representative may be made from a different point of view. When we oppose such a term as 'rhythmic' to representative, implying thereby that what is rhythmic does not represent, we ought to raise for ourselves the doubt, ought we not ? whether rhythm in art may not, after all, be indeed a representation of natural rhythm like walking and running, like the beat of a horse's hoofs, or like the eternal monotony of the waves of the sea. Or, again, if we use the term, formal, in the same way, are there not abstract forms in nature like the circle of the horizon or the apparent vault of the heavens ? And might not, therefore, the ' formal ' quality of a picture turn out to be a kind of ' representation ' of such abstract form ?

Botticelli, for example, had a singular gift for painting round pictures. There is no doubt that the peculiar beauty of the *tondo* known as the Madonna of the Magnificat depends upon the general harmony of the things represented in that picture with its circular form. And, after all, mày not the subtlety of this harmony be really due to a concealed resemblance to abstract forms that have no intelligible relation to what the picture portends to be ' about ' ?

It is very necessary that we should take full account of this difficulty. It is one the burden of which we must carry with us yet for a considerable time ; but let us note here and now one very definite answer to it. It is that even in a picture whose main intention is very clearly the representation of natural objects, landscape or human faces or the movement and action of a battle-field, this immediately representative tendency is held in very severe limitation by the sensibility of the artist for abstract form which goes to negate the immediately representative intention. Now, if we are to call the formal aspect of such a picture the ' representation ' of some abstract form in nature, such representation is of a very obscure and doubtful kind compared with the unmistakeable desire to render something of the real landscape or the human faces which we suppose to fascinate the painter. The very most that can be said is that *if* qualities of form can indeed be traced to an obscure or unrecognised tendency towards representation on the part of the painter, that obscure tendency operates in a direction that diverges entirely from the obvious or conscious representative character of the picture. If, on the contrary, the sources of form and rhythm in pictorial art are *not* to be traced back merely to unrecognised representation, there still remains the opposition between the painter's intention to represent something and his sensibility to values other than representative.

In view of this divergence, we shall continue to speak of representative and rhythmic or formal qualities, and to speak of them in opposition. As we proceed with our analysis, we shall find, I think, that we do not need to go back upon our footsteps ; and that the antithesis can be grounded in ultimate psychological fact.

Nevertheless we must be prepared also to find that the transition from the representative to the formal in art, or the relation that holds between them, states one of the hardest problems of æsthetic. It is perhaps the crux of the whole science. But in this very difficulty, I should urge, there lies the psychological and philosophical value of the distinction in question. At no point so much as in this very discussion of representative *versus* non-representative art is it so easy to fall into an arid or even sterile dialectic that lets the real experience slip away altogether and leads nowhere. The difficulty is one inherent in æsthetic. It is that of not allowing one's sensibility to the many-sidedness of the world of art to become ungenuine and devitalised, and at the same time, of not departing from the sincerity of a rigorous philosophical dialectic. I do not know that there is anyone in the history of æsthetic theory who achieves this which such complete success as Schopenhauer.

Schopenhauer in his treatment of the æsthetic side of his problem shows a profound sensibility to the distinction between the arts that are characteristically representative and those that are not. Yet his classification of the arts was by no means that of the representative *versus* the non-representative. It could not be, because architecture is placed along with painting and sculpture in their opposition to music.

What Schopenhauer does is simply to divide the world of art into two by placing music on one side and by opposing it to all the other arts.

This division of the arts and the exaltation of music to an altogether unique position among them has been condemned as arbitrary, or even fantastic. But Schopenhauer's real intention is clear—to exhibit the special æsthetic qualities of music through its dominantly formal and non-representative character. It was as non-representative that he conceived it to possess the unique power over human sensibility with which he invested it. For he thought of it, as in some way an analogue or typification of the will or universal life-force ; and this in its very nature was incapable of any kind of pictorial representation. The negation of representative possibilities, therefore, in music becomes a key to its peculiar values.

The difficulty we must now encounter is that our initial method of approach to art is not so serviceable in the case of music. For when we consider the beauty of pure music without the voice, or of quasi-geometrical design and of all that we can bring under that term, it has no apparent meaning to say that in such kind of beauty the artist is looking at nature through a medium. When we thought of the painter as looking at nature through his medium, the expression was not metaphorical at least in so far as the idea of vision does actually mean that he sees the landscape with the bodily eye. The sculptor does actually see, and must see, the living bodies of the men and women that are the objects he is striving to delineate. The poet does actually see the faces and gauge the expression of the men and women who, albeit through the transfiguration that poetry effects, do nevertheless enter into the poem. And this is true on the most formal view that can be taken of these arts. It might, I think, be summarised or typified or drawn to a focus through the emphasis that Mr. Laurence Binyon, in his contrast between the art of the East and the art of the West, places upon "that concentrated attention on the human form which is at the core of Western painting."[1]

There is no corresponding real, natural object that the composer of pure instrumental music can be said, in any literal sense, to see, or to perceive with any sense organ. Or again, beyond the abstract lines of the arch of Norman or early English Gothic, no natural object can be conceived to lie, or to possess the builder's attention through any avenue of sense. If it be granted that the pointed arch is a phallic symbol, or is like a lancet or a leaf form ; or that the round arch is like the rising sun, these associations are, at the most, indefinitely remote. It would be absurd to speak of lancets or leaves as constituting the goal of a "concentrated attention" on the part of the builder, in the sense in which Mr. Binyon speaks of the human body in relation to the Western painter.

Since this is so clearly and manifestly true, might not the entire validity of our method of approach to art be called in question ? Just because it appears to be of such partial application, would it not follow that it has no general or philosophical significance whatever ? That conclusion could, or indeed must, be drawn, unless some real continuity be shown between the most representative arts, like painting, and the most formal or rhythmical like architecture or music, in respect of the application of our method. This continuity, I think, can certainly be exhibited. It is important, however, first to stress the aspect of dis-continuity which we are now encountering between art in its representative tendency and art in its non-representative and formal character.

What, therefore, we have now to observe is the gradual transformation or modification that our

[1] *Painting in the Far East*, by Lawrence Binyon, p. 112.

formula, 'plasticity and vision,' will undergo as we apply it through types of art of ever decreasing representative intention. What will happen to it, we might ask, when, in the end, we make it try to bridge the gulf between, *e.g.*, the most realistic painting, and the most formal of pure non-vocal music ?

(2)

When the painter brings up his medium to his view of the object, he begins to see it, in some way, different from the ' real ' external object. He may, or he may not, recognise this difference. What is important for our purpose is the degree of his absorption in the contemplation of the object. Through the plasticity of his medium, mere sight is changed into vision—a vision that is necessarily different from perception.

The artist, however, need not, and perhaps often does not, know that the things he ' sees ' in the object do not really belong to it. His absorption in the object will in any case be deepened in proportion to the deepening interest of the things he ' sees ' in it ; and such an absorbing and ever-increasing interest may affect him in many different ways with regard to the handling of his medium. He may, for example, fancy the object to be so interesting that the medium he has begun with is not sufficiently transparent to reveal the complex character of the object, or not sufficiently brilliant to show up its glowing lights. The history of art, both in art tradition and individual artistic development, is full of attempts to find, for example, media that can more realistically delineate the object. This was very largely the tendency of mediæval painting as it developed, say, from the twelfth or thirteenth century to the seventeenth. Even granting—as so much modern criticism contends —that it was a decadent movement, it is nevertheless a matter of historical and psychological fact. It expresses an intention that appears, in some way, in the history of art in every country and in every race.

Yet, however intent the artist may be upon a realistic aim, the time must come sooner or later, when he recognises that his work is different from the object in some essential respect. This felt difference from the object may, again, have very varying effects upon the artist. One effect might be to make him feel dissatisfied with his work because it seemed to diverge so far from the appearance of the object. But another effect has sometimes been to convince the artist that with this difference there is bound up an essential element of beauty. The work is *not* like nature and *yet* it is beautiful *in virtue of* its very departure from nature.

At first sight this departure from nature might be supposed to express itself along two very different lines. It might express itself along the line which we have been trying to interpret through the idea of projection of the unconscious. In so far, however, as this means that the artist ' sees ' in the object things that are not ' really ' there, it is a departure that need by no means run counter to a representative intention. He may just as well, and just as easily, ' represent ' things that are not really there as things that are, so long as what he ' represents ' can be expressed in ' representative ' terms. This only means, for example, that the novelist who takes some real woman as the point of origin of his heroine is at full artistic liberty to make a blend of her either with some other ' real ' lady or with the lady of his own mind. In so far as all three women in question are ' Nature,' they may be portrayed in a naturalistic intention. Projection of the unconscious—*la donna della sua mente*—does not in itself seem to involve any considerable departure from naturalism, and from 'naturalism' in a sense in which it is almost equivalent to realism. At all events, *if* it does, the necessity by which it does so involve a non-realistic movement has not yet emerged along the lines of our argument.

We must, therefore, look for the real line of departure from naturalism or realism at the point where the artist, though intent upon some realistic aim, recognises the value of form—of something that is essentially divergent from his realistic intention, and yet surprises him with its beauty—of something that is essentially different from anything that ever was on land or sea and yet that imparts a transcendental beauty to his mountains and his ocean.

It may very well be that some artists have painted or chiselled without realising this essential departure from the mere delineation of the object. In general, however, it will not be so. To some extent even those artists working in the most apparently realistic intention will be conscious of the need for departure from likeness to the object, and of the value that this departure implies. Suppose, then, that an artist becomes deeply conscious of the beauty of that element that is divergent from his realistic aim, again, it will affect him through his medium—whether in his choice of other possible media, or through his handling of the one by which he happens to have made the discovery. Here, then, the general line of his interest in the object has undergone deflection, whether transitory, or more than transitory. His interest has flowed, for the moment at least, into something that he recognises as different from the object ; and it may further come about that in this difference he has become consciously interested.

He may perceive that much more might be made of this divergence. His aim, therefore, is no longer so purely to see the object. It has become the desire at least to retain that aspect of the 'vision' which he knows to be out of accord with the 'reality.' But perhaps it is a little more than even that. Perhaps it has become transformed into the desire to unearth the new element of beauty by still further emphasising the unlikeness of his 'vision' to the 'reality.' Now it is quite possible that he may do this by changing, a little, the way in which he moulds his plastic material; but it may equally well be that he thinks of trying another kind of medium altogether—a medium that may better serve to bring out the difference between his 'vision' of the object at this point from the known 'reality.' That is to say, it may be in his option to choose a medium, which in the specific intention of the moment, will be relatively less transparent than the one he has been using.

In order to employ the terms, transparent and opaque, in their literal sense, let us move out of the realm of art for a moment ; and think simply of the interposition between the eye and an object of planes of translucent material that can have different degrees of transparency and opacity. Colourless plate glass will give a very different impression ; etched glass still another, and so on. Each kind of glass will have its own effect in relation to the unconscious. When we look at an eclipse of the sun through smoked glass, we cannot help the feeling of loneliness and awe that comes over us in such a black and empty universe with its single piercing and melancholy light, though we know we are not really more alone than before.

Returning to the realm of art with this analogy in our mind, though we cannot, except in a few rare[1] cases, use the terms, transparent and opaque in any very literal sense, we must nevertheless be fully alive

[1] The actual 'vision' of the heavens that one has through the transparent windows of Chartres Cathedral is, of course, a very important case.

to the significance of a medium that seems to relate the eye or the ear very immediately to the object— ' the bit of nature '—and to the significance of one that seems to blur the object rather than to show it up clearly. There are media that seem to be relatively ' transparent ' to the object ; and media that seem to be relatively ' opaque.' Fresco seems to be, in however small a degree, inherently more opaque than oils. One must always take pleasure in the exquisite blurring of its outlines. Of course, there may be realistic fresco and impressionist, post- or super-impressionist painting ; but that does not affect the essentials of the argument.

The artist, then, thus in quest of new possibilities, may take refuge in some other and relatively more opaque medium. That is to say, his aim as regards the object has altered a little. He has become willing to obscure it to some extent, or to shut out some of its aspects. Just as in his ' vision ' of the object, he need not know to what extent he is ' seeing ' things that are not there ; so now in the new phase of his work, he need not know to what extent he is shutting out the object, or veiling certain of its aspects. He need not know how far he is blurring its outlines or fusing its colours. Of course, he *may* know and he may desire to investigate. Most probably there will always be some knowledge and some ignorance.

It is the blurring of the object and the fusing of its colours through the increasing opacity of the medium that become our means of introduction to a new aspect of art ; to something that will help us towards a revision of our initial standpoint. Take, first, a case where we can apply the terms ' blurring ' and ' fusing ' in a literal sense. In a portrait, the face and the upper part of the dress may be drawn with extreme clearness—with a certain unmistakeable definiteness of representative intention. But the

lower part of the bust need not so be drawn. It may
fade by imperceptible degrees into the darkness and
obscurity of the background. Yet we know that the
dress on the living person could have been discerned
with a continuous clearness. This is the art of the
portrait painter, to balance the obscurity of the
background against the distinctness of the features,
and to secure the balance without violence of contrast
and by imperceptible gradation. This is the formal
or rhythmical aspect of the portrait—the balance,
and the mode by which the balancing is effected, of
background with features. It is the rhythm of
darkness and light. Goethe, in speaking of Scott's
description of Ivanhoe's dress as he enters the hall of
Cedric in the deepening twilight, remarks that it was
a fault to mention that the Palmer wore sandals. The
attention of the reader is directed to the feet which,
in the semi-darkness of the torch-light, could not be
seen. " Daylight enters at once," Goethe observes.
Or, in other words, Scott's realism was at variance
with his sense of form. It was more important that
the sense of darkness should be emotionally or
rhythmically communicated than that the detail—
in itself interesting—should be introduced. Scott's
exact, scientific or antiquarian genius, had, for the
moment, got above the artistic.

It thus seems as if the idea of form and rhythm
in art were going to emerge through the conception
of a medium that tends to obscure rather than to
reveal. We shall see by and by how this aspect of the
matter is emphasised through consideration of the
art of music. It is music that will raise the question
of form with inevitable challenge and state the problem
with a special definiteness.

Meantime we have to remark that shutting out or
obscuring nature is a negative conception ; and it
cannot easily be conceived that an artist will work

in an orientation that has no other essential character
save this negative one. We must, therefore, look for
its positive side. The cue might, I think, be found
in some such analogy as that of Milton's blindness.
It is quite certain that in the invocation to light,

> thou
> Revisit'st not these eyes, that rowle in vain
> To find thy piercing ray, and find no dawn;
> So thick a drop serene hath quench'd thir Orbs
> Or dim suffusion veil'd—

the poet is not merely uttering a complaint, but is also
achieving a profound acquiescence—an acquiescence
that has a note of austere triumph in it because of the
new powers which it is to reveal in himself. The
darkness is something that compels him to discover
within, what he might never otherwise have found,
or found to less advantage and value.

> Yet not the more
> Cease I to wander where the Muses haunt . . .
> So much the rather thou Celestial light
> Shine inward.

It is noteworthy, too, that in this very passage, specific
mention is made of the formal aspect of his art ; and
it is spoken of as if it came directly from the inward
meditation enforced upon him by his blindness.

> Chief
> Thee *Sion* and the flowrie brooks beneath
> That wash thy hallowed feet and warbling flow
> Nightly I visit ; nor sometimes forget
> Those other two equal'd with me in Fate
> So were I equal'd with them in renown,
> Blind *Thamyris* and blind *Maeonides*
> And *Tiresias* and *Phineus* Prophets old.
> Then feed on thoughts, that voluntarie move
> Harmonious numbers . . .

Of course, we do not go to a poet in his poetry—least
of all to Milton—for philosophic reflection about his
work. The passage none the less serves as a somewhat
startling and unexpected illustration of the view that
I am trying meanwhile to shape in outline. Just as
the shutting out of the bright world of sense is a nega-

tive condition of those thoughts "that voluntarie move harmonious numbers," so, in terms of our general conception, the partial shutting out of the natural object through the relative obscurity of the medium is a negative condition of a more inward orientation of the artist. With the emergence of form, or as an implication of that, he cannot, or cannot so easily, look outward, and must, therefore, in some senes, look within.

(3)

What are the conditions which, in art, go most in the direction of shutting out the natural world, with its discreet and tangible objects of perception—the men and women who live in it, their individual bodies and their characteristic gestures that so thrust upon us the individuality of life and soul that they express ? Architecture and music may surely be taken as going much further than painting in this direction of concealing or veiling nature in so far as nature means outer objects and the concrete in-dividualities of living organisms. Music, however, partly because of its great range and variety, partly because of its intensive qualities, offers us a peculiarly valuable field within which to work out the point now at issue.

In regard to the evolution of music, two things need to be kept well in view. These are its origins in song, on the one hand, and in dancing, on the other. Of these two points of origin, however, one is more important than the other. Song is more inherently and vitally pervasive of music through all stages of its history than dancing. All music retains in some degree the qualities of melody ; and melody in whatever form, is always immediately and in-timately reminiscent of song. There are some kinds

135

of music, such as the early music of the Latin church that have moved very far away from the rhythms of the dance. In so far, therefore, as music is limited and controlled through its two points of origin, we must look for a very much more immediate limitation through singing than through dancing.

The voice, in music, cannot as a rule be used without words. It is true that crooning has a certain peculiar effect of its own ; and we must not forget the strange and mystical effect of the voices, employed without words and just as instruments of the orchestra, in Scriabin's *Prometheus*.

But as a rule, vocal music is burdened, as it were, with the intelligible and representative power of words. This links it up with poetry as an art that has—ostensibly, at least—something to tell you about. Vocal music, however, is far more remote from the objects about which it tells you than poetry ; or at all events, it tells you about it with far less intellectual distinctness.

Further, there is, on the whole, an immense difference between the effect of song and the effect of pure instrumental music. When music is being played, and the chorus suddenly bursts in, it creates a new and specifically different attitude on the part of the listener. When they begin to sing, even though you cannot catch a word of what they are singing about, you know they are telling you something ; and the manner of your receptiveness and sensibility is deeply changed.

We should be able to trace, in another way, the nature of this change through the historical development of music as it freed itself from words and the burden of their intellectual content. This is a very instructive case of the transition from an art which tells you *about* something to one which apparently has no object to tell about.

TRANSITION TO MUSIC

This point needs to be worked out with care. For we have to notice that where music is sung, the words that are sung give, or may give, the greater part of the representative content. Merely, therefore, by playing on an instrument or instruments, music originally intended to be sung, we might achieve a very complete *saltus* from an æsthetic effect with a full or obvious representative content to one of a more purely formal and non-representative character. I suppose this is, on the whole, true of the earlier instrumental music in Europe. To illustrate from a source by no means the earliest, but serviceable to us now because of its familiarity—Bach's organ music is often very close to the chorale in general character. But its qualities of form are achieved not so much along the line of any evolution of form, as merely by dropping the medium—i.e., words—that originally carried the greater burden of representative significance. It is only later on, in the Romantic period, say roughly from Beethoven's Pastoral Symphony to Strauss' Alpine Symphony that pure instrumental music is striving to get back representative values in a new direction.

Almost every statement here needs to be made with reservation. For, of course, Bach is constantly striving after representative effects, as for example— to take an instance of extraordinary naïveté—when he makes the bass *fall a seventh* in the Chorale-Prelude, " In Adam's Fall." And again, the Strauss symphony that gives such a wonderfully realistic ' vision ' of the Alpine landscape does so without at all violating the natural laws of our sensibility to pure music. But with all the reservations that have to be made, and allowing for the ever-changing and ever-alternating movements, now towards representative content, and now away from it, there is a tremendous cleavage, a real transition εἰs ἄλλο γένos, as

we pass from song to non-vocal music.   In especial,
I think it is in the great period of instrumental music,
say from Bach to Mozart, that we should look for
those types of work that most fully and unambiguously
illustrate the qualities of music on the side of the
perfection of its form and rhythm.

There is a metaphor that I should like to employ
at this point.   It is that of the watershed.   As
historically the voice was withdrawn from music, we
might mark in this historical transition a crossing of
the watershed between the arts of representation and
the arts of rhythm.   The relation of the singing voice
to the instrument should, therefore, be a mode of
differentiation—a kind of touchstone, discriminating
the line of what is perhaps the greatest cleavage in
the universe of art.   I mean that though we have to
look for continuity everywhere, there is nevertheless
a native and ineradicable tendency in music to
decide either one way or the other, to be specifically
vocal and representative, or specifically non-vocal or
non-representative—to fall, that is to say, either to
one or other side of the watershed.

In all ordinary forms of music, of course, like the
mass or the opera, the vocal is continually alternating
with the instrumental.   But the impressiveness of
the alternation is perhaps explicable through the
tendency of music to become specific, one way or the
other.   And then, almost all accompanied vocal
music is interspersed—begun or concluded—with
instrumental sound alone.   This perhaps emphasises
the fact that because it *is* music with which we are
dealing, it must finally differentiate itself as abstract
sound distinct from singing.

What happens then, exactly, when the voice is
withdrawn from music ?

Like architecture on the side of its architectonic
or general formal quality, music on the side of its

rhythmic quality becomes a medium of reflection for the artist's own mind rather than a medium of relationship of that mind to other objects. The characteristic forms that emerge in architecture are not like things in the natural and spatial world. Nor in music are the characteristic forms that emerge in its temporal progression at all like the forms that usually belong to nature, whether to nature, as expressed in a temporal series or as expressed in space. Music is, in general, representative neither of things visible and permanent, nor yet of things audible and taking place in time, as, for example, the sound of flowing waters, or of thunder or tempest, or even of human speech or the song of birds. Music is far more closely akin to the mathematical and the symmetrical in so far as these may be thought as a time series and expressed in a temporal rhythm. And it is because the nature of the medium—musical sound—resists with more or less vigour any approximation to natural sounds, or to intelligible sounds, like human speech, that it forms such a splendid and unique means of self-reflection for the artist. Sound—the ordered sound of musical tones—the simple scale of which has so definite a mathematical arrangement, and the combinations and relations of whose tones present a form that can be best described through mathematical analogy, has become a medium not so much in the sense that it mediates anything to the creative or receptive mind, as in the sense that it mediates a certain movement of that mind with itself, or becomes the means of a new self-relation. If, therefore, we might re-adapt the old formula in which we regarded the medium as standing between, and bringing together, the artist and his object, we might say now that in music musical sound is what mediates the artist to himself. In such a re-adaptation, we preserve the concept of plasticity ; but vision, in so far as it has necessarily come to signify ' inward vision,' tends also to be denuded of all save its analogical content.

Take the case of Wagner who was most deeply interested in the synthesis of the other arts with music, and who strove so hard for a real marriage of the arts of colour and form, and of the art of poetry, with music. Why is it that he instinctively withdraws everything that the voice can give or that the eye can receive at certain passages of his music where his intention is clearly that the tragic effect should be supreme ? Of course, he is only following the line of an already long established tradition that gives the orchestra its position of lonely glory over and above the dramatic action as presented on the stage and rendered by the voices. But in those wonderful commentaries of his, those majestic, brooding reflections upon the action that are played by the orchestra when the curtain is down and the theatre is in darkness, there is a deliberate intention of absorption in sound alone, of concentration within the experiencing soul itself, that necessitates the exclusion alike of intelligible words and of visible forms. I incline to think that the orchestral commentaries in *Parsifal* or in *The Ring* show this intention in its highest achievement ; and for my own part I know of nothing in art where, for a few moments, there is felt such a tremendous concentration of an inwardly directed energy, such a complete absorption of the experiencing soul in itself, as in Siegfried's Funeral March in the *Götterdämmerung*. It gives us the most absolute, the most unimpaired example of the tragic spirit.

In such passages, then, the medium of the art seems rather to exclude or to veil whatsoever we may regard as the object of the artist's vision ' To veil ' is perhaps better than ' to exclude ' ; and even so, we must not consider the veiling as absolute or total. However inward be the nature of the experience, or to however great an extent the imaginative forms demanded by the medium tend to negate relationship with outer objects, the world lying beyond is never quite concealed or shut out. The reader may remember that in a previous chapter when we first touched upon the nature of the tragic spirit, we supposed that the object upon which the artist 'projected' the content of his unconscious might be called 'the suffering of the world.' He could not do this, it seemed, without in some way depriving that suffering of its absoluteness, of its sheer reality of fact. Here, since we are dealing with Wagner and with Wagner's effort to get at the deepest lying emotions of life, we might call the object that he seems to keep in view 'the primeval universe,' or something like that. In order, however, to be able to project his own primeval or archetypal imagination upon it, here, too, he cannot deal with it in its absoluteness. He must deprive it of something ; he must deprive it of its own terrible reality, existence and life ; and this he can do through the magnificent rhythms and abstract forms of music. Sound is the veil which stands between him and the primeval universe ; it cannot altogether conceal it ; the veil is not quite impenetrable ; but it is impenetrable to the extent of throwing Wagner back upon himself and making him go down into the depths of himself, thus effecting a self-mediation that is largely, though never entirely, independent of the primeval reality that lies beyond the medium. The moment of self-mediation is, in the totality of the experience, greater than the moment of mediation to the object beyond. This is the essential of the tragic spirit.

In so far, however, as I had before to grant that 'vision' in such types of music is denuded of all save its analogical content, I may now safely make the reservation that something objective is still sensuously apprehended, though the degree of that objective apprehension may be exceedingly low, or at a vanishing point.

We have now to examine in yet a little further detail the nature of musical sound as a medium of art before we can do entire justice to Schopenhauer's philosophical intention.

(4)

The remarkable thing about the art of music in its evolution is the very great length of time before it really came to its own. For hundreds of years, it was little more than the experimenting of choristers singing together separate parts to form a pleasurable sound. It came quite suddenly at last, issuing in the discovery of counterpoint and harmony. But so far as the modern world is concerned, the medium of music was not known, was not to hand, until this had been done. That is to say, by a rough contrast of the arts of sculpture and music, the clay or the marble was given by earth ready to hand ; whereas the medium of music took the labour of many generations to evolve.

Note first, however, that if we compare vocal music with sculpture, this contrast does not hold, or does not hold so closely. For the vocal chords are a natural medium ready to hand, not certainly in the sense in which clay is ready to hand, but in the sense, at least, in which language is ready to hand. But instrumental music as the matter of enormous cultural significance that we recognise it to have been in Europe, could not practically begin until there was some sort of a system of counterpoint. And the evolution of that took, as we remarked, generations numbered at least in tens.

Correlated, perhaps, to this is the other significant

fact that when you come to the medium of music you do not feel your fingers in contact with some earthy (or fleshly) stuff as you do in the case of all the other arts, sculpture, architecture, painting, dancing, vocal music, and—more doubtfully—poetry. What you really feel them in contact with is the wood or metal or ivory. None of these is earthy in the feel of them. They have no doubt grown out of the earth, or been dug out of it ; but the gnomes and brownies have been at work for years long in mine and forest before you can get them. There is another significant fact, too, about music. You must somehow contrive to set the air vibrating, in a very palpable way. This, too, you often have to do with your lungs and lips. Trying to generalise, the instrumental musician's medium is air driven through pipes of wood and metal. But the varieties are too manifold and too nice to admit of easy generalisation. Significant, for example, is the magnificent command of the organist through his feet upon bars of wood, of an underworld of voluminous and palpable darkness. And then, too, it might just as well be said that the true medium of the musician is a pen and ink and ledger-lined paper. So it is, and the significance of the fact is made clear by Beethoven's warning to young composers that they must learn to write without the pianoforte—advice he could not himself always follow, or did not always choose to follow. Further, this power of the composer to write alone in his room pre-supposes all the labour of the generations of experimenting monks. What is the medium then ? The paper and ink, or the wind and wood and metal ?

An obvious answer would be that the attitude of the composer (the creative artist) to his art cannot be the same as that of the player (the interpretive artist). Every difference in the attitude of the artist implies a correlative difference in the medium employed. But

there is, it seems to me, an answer of a more general
and comprehensive character.

The medium of the musician is wood and metal
rather than earth or stone. These are not given like
earth. Wood grows in the forest and is hewn by
human labour. Metal is smelted from the ore by
human labour. Sculpture in marble and the music of
the orchestra stand, therefore, in a curious contrast in
respect of their media. Wood-carving and the casting
of bronze offer a kind of middle term and prevent our
taking the contrast too absolutely. Nevertheless let
us consider the contrast as it presents itself, sufficiently
significant. The sculptor stands *vis-à-vis* his block of
marble, a bit of earth unaltered by the forces either of
nature or of man. The musician's contact with the
earth is less close by several removes. There intervene
both man and nature. The marble, or its texture,
was never devised by any mind to meet any human
need. In its veining we can trace no operative
purpose, conscious or unconscious. The marble is just
there, and to this absolute environment containing
no embodiment, no record, no imprint, of any life or
experience, the sculptor must respond in a relation of
sheer immediacy. The relation of the musician to the
musical instrument is quite different. Correlated to
the evolution of the tonal system through many
generations is the evolution of the *organon* through
which that system can at any time be interpreted or
actualised. On the one side, there are the generations
of experimenting choristers. On the other, there is
the system of adaptation which leads from the mine
and the forests up to the finished *organon*. The
musician's relation, therefore, to his *organon* is
mediated in a two-fold way—from without and from
within. It is mediated from without because the
labour of the gnomes and cabires of the Teutonic
North is conditioned by, and responds to, the travail

of the mediæval singers of the Italian South. It is mediated from within, because the musician's sensibility to sound is based upon the evolution of the tonal system he has inherited from them all. But, it will be asked, does not the sculptor, too, inherit from his past the discoveries of an earlier age ? He does. But the mode of his inheritance is specifically different. His inheritance, whatever it is, whether transmitted at birth, or acquired through cultural tradition, is *all* within himself. On the other hand, for the musician, the medium is already rich with the imprints of human experience. You cannot *touch*—let alone play upon— any instrument that adequately embodies our modern tonal system without overwhelming yourself in a flood of ancient memories., Play the simplest progression in music—the plagal or the authentic cadence —and you build up cathedral walls about you in spite of yourself. That is why the medium, in this art, seems to have a certain pre-eminence over the media of other arts. It *implies* so much. So much is enfolded within it. And that is why music, as an art, is such a superb instrument of the human spirit. The musician is compelled to embody so much of the experience of his race.

But, it will be said again, is not poetry like music in respect of its medium ? Has not human speech been the product of a long evolution and does not it, too, embody the experience of countless generations within its structure ? In so far as language is the product of an evolution, it has the same kind of difference from marble that the medium of music has. But then, language is almost purely the work of nature, and in forming it the conscious purpose of man comes in hardly at all. The part played by scholar and lexicographer in the evolution of language is almost negligible. All they do is just to effect one or two little finishing touches to the product already completed in all essential respects. Not so with the experimenting choristers. Before they began there was no medium—or only something that the modern world would have found incredibly rudimentary and insufficient. So that they literally and consciously co-operate with nature in the evolution of the medium in a fashion that has no parallel in the natural evolution of a language. Therefore, the natural voice of poetry *in respect of its medium* is a voice that comes much more directly from the earth than the voice of music does in respect of its medium. When the lips speak, they set in motion the waves of the surrounding air unconsciously, nor need there be now, or ever have been, any consciousness of what they do. When the musician sets a-vibrating his columns of air he feels, he almost touches, the informing spirit of the moving wind. And the enclosed spaces within which he makes it vibrate are given him through the long travail of the human mind, working quite consciously. How did that curiously shaped enclosed space that makes violin music come to be devised as of just that shape ?

The problem of music with respect to its medium may indeed be said to be the plasticity of the moving wind. That is what makes the voice of music such an ethereal voice, and in a sense, so unearthly.

When, therefore, we go back to the question with which this digression began : Is the medium of the musician metal and wood and wind, or is it just ledger-lined paper in the composer's quiet study ? we begin to see that it does not really matter along which line of thought we move. For in any case, the musician is confronted not with a bare material, but with a material which already contains the deep imprints of ages of human experience. Contrast, therefore, the poet in his quiet, lonely room and the composer in his. Before the one the paper is blank—

a pure white. Before the other it lies covered with groups of five parallel lines ; and therein is all the difference. These lines are *engrams* of the experience of the generations, written not in the artist's mind, or not in that alone, but in the material thing that lies before his eye and hand.

That is why music—so it seems to me—sweeps up within its movement more of the past experience of humanity than any other art can do. It is the nature of its medium to embody the immediate past of our race—that past, namely, during which the medium was itself undergoing its evolution and perfection, a past, say roughly of a thousand years, or at least, not more than two thousand. But, then, if music is thus placed in a position of advantage with respect to the immediate past, we might conceive also that this advantage would be of avail also with respect to the more remote past. When the immediate past is called forth by any means, it seems not unlikely that it will be in close association with the remote past, or that the two will blend and come forth together. In other words, we may conceive that music is, of all the arts, able to reach the deepest-lying of the archetypes, or to reach the archetypes at their deepest level. This, I think, is what Schopenhauer meant when he emphasised that quality of music which can best be described as depth.

The difference between music and the other arts in this respect, is, of course, not absolute. It would not justify the *absoluteness* of the cleavage which Schopenhauer asserts to hold good in the world of art. Nevertheless, the difference, relative as it may be, is so striking—at points so nearly complete— that it is worth our while to dwell upon it a little. It will serve, in especial, to make clear certain things with regard to individual attitude and social relations in art.

ART AND THE UNCONSCIOUS

In so far as we suppose the experience of past generations to be embodied in the tonal system which constitutes the medium of music, the artist, as composer, is thereby rendered at once more independent of his external world, and at the same time placed in a new relation of dependence upon it in another way.

He is rendered more independent of it, because, as we saw, his medium does not so much relate him to outer objects as gives him a new means of relating him to himself. And we may suppose, or rather I should say, we may legitimately infer, that musical sound forms so splendid a means of self-relation, or of self-interpretation just because of the human experience—the experience of past generations—that it contains, so to speak, in the form of potential energy. The composer need not use it so much as a means of seeing the natural or human world that lies beyond it as of finding the reflection of his own mind in the very experience which it contains. Pure music would, therefore, be the most inward form of art, that form in which the artist is most freed from the dominance of outward things, which gives the most security for the deep apprehension of the mind by itself, and which offers the greatest possibilities of inward harmony and oneness of the soul with itself. Whether it would be legitimate to say that for us in the West, it offers the best means for that kind of self-apprehension and self-unity that the East secures through its profounder religious experience, I hesitate to decide. But I suggest that it is in music that the religious experience of our Western world has most nearly come to its own and has achieved what its religion without music would never have achieved.

And so if I accept the definition of the tragic spirit in art, as that aspect of beauty, which depends for its fulness most entirely on the self-relation and self-unity of the mind, and least of all, upon rapport with external objects, I should take pure instrumental music as that type of art which gives the best rendering of the spirit of tragedy. We shall see, later on, how this conclusion will have to be modified in the light of such a movement as the English drama in the time of Elizabeth. But even so, I think, we shall be able to bring it into relation with such facts without altering it in essential respects.

Secondly, and not so much in opposition to, as in correlation with, the fact of the inwardness of music, there must be taken into account also the extraordinary dependence of the musician upon his outer world. The ledger lines on the paper—the paper that for the literary artist is a mere blank—represent not only the imprints of the past in the composer's medium; they imply also a subtlety and complexity of social relations not elsewhere found to the same extent in the world of art. It has been well said that the massiveness of stone involves the architect in a relation of dependence upon the financial and economic functions of society to an extent scarcely exhibited in any other form of art.[1] The fact that music always has such an imperative need of the interpreter is one of the most characteristic features of the art. Interpretation, in music, does in fact hold a position between the creativeness of the composer and the appreciation of the audience that finds no exact counterpart in any other sphere of art, perhaps not even in the drama.

Hence not so much in spite, as in virtue, of its inward character music is also, in this relation, the most social of the arts. Generalising a little at this point, and speaking in the widest sense of ' the spirit of tragedy,' we have to note that the tragic spirit is at once the most inward and the most social of all the forms of artistic experience. This is important from the religious point of view. It is the essence of

---

[1] Cf. Edward Bullough : *Mind and Medium in Art*, p. 33.

religion to be inward, and it is also essential that it should be social.

In the antique world, the Attic drama fulfilled these conditions to as great an extent as was perhaps possible in Europe. In modern times, it is pure music, or music that approximates to the type of pure music, that most effectually performs in art, this function of at once expressing the most inward needs of the soul, and of doing it in such a way as to bring into prominence the essentially social movement in this very inwardness itself.

In Bach's organ music, in the Mass in B minor, in certain passages in Wagner's Tetralogy or in *Parsifal*, this strange correlation of inwardness and social unity is rendered in a way that is most integral with, and that perhaps does most honour to, the essentials of Western culture.

CHAPTER VI

ART AS THE RELATION OF OUTER AND INNER

To speak of things in abstract and general terms is always dangerous. But here I cannot refrain from saying that the West is *extension*, the East is *intension*.

YU-LAN FUNG
(*International Journal of Ethics*, April, 1922)

Every self is a copula, a meeting-point of tension and fulfilment,
a self-maintenance of the one life through a portion of the external,
and of the external as centred in a case of the one life. But, as it is
distinctly figured in the poem, the complete experience brings together
all the selves, with nothing omitted, but transfigured and expanded
by the place they hold and the illumination they receive in it. . . .
The selves who figure in the poem have all rendered up their content
to the great experience which was the poet's mind.

BOSANQUET, of *The Divina Comedia*

(1)

THE words, East and West, have sometimes been
used in the development of our subject as expressive
of different and antithetical attitudes to life. It may
be easy, no doubt, to exaggerate the difference
implied ; and it would be well, therefore, when we
thus play off the two terms against each other, to
accept them as symbolical or emblematic ; as indi-
cative, that is to say, of tendency, rather than as
assertive of absolute fact. Nevertheless such safeguard must not be taken to imply that the divergence
in tendency, whatever it is, is not of the utmost
significance. Napoleon and Buddha stand for differences of as great an import as can anywhere be found
in life and experience.

The words, outer and inner, too, have been freely
used. Nor have they been used without the assump-

tion that they characterise the attitudes or tendencies thus attributed to West and East. Again, whatever safeguards one may feel bound to make against absoluteness of assertion, they must stop short of denying the inwardness of the genius of the East, and the relative outwardness of that of the West, or of lessening the sense of reality involved in the contrast.

The term, outer, however, has, for our subject, a very definite literal or spatial application. When it is said, for example, that a man looks outward, it means, or may mean, that he does in fact see things that lie beyond the periphery of his body. It may, of course, mean more than this, and be taken to imply that he is in search of things not immediately visible or even that may never become accessible to sense. It is nevertheless capable of the most literal application. On the other hand, when it is said that a man looks inward, it does not seem clear what meaning can be attributed to it if any emphasis is laid upon its literal or spatial significance. Usually, the phrase, ' looking inward,' is taken to mean a metaphorical extension of an idea, originally used of the spatial world, into a domain whose nature it is no longer possible to conceive according to spatial laws. There is a danger, however, in admitting too readily that the spatial implications must altogether be renounced, or that the expression has become a mere metaphor. For negatively, the inward orientation is defined through the closing of the avenues of sense by which outward things, in the literal meaning, may make their impression upon the mind. The exclusion of outward things, therefore, in the literal sense, thus conditions the inward orientation. Beyond this negative limitation, however, it is not easy to find a positive meaning in the idea of, for example, inward vision, in so far as ' inward ' should be taken to imply, ' spatially inward.' Perhaps it can be done ;

but it is at all events not a perfectly simple or obvious matter.

The difficulty of extending the spatial implication of the word, inward, has an important bearing upon art ; or, at all events, makes an important suggestion. It is always much easier to describe the outward orientation of art. ' Outward ' may not, indeed, be always taken literally any more than ' inward ' ; but it begins in a literal application to space, and it is fairly easy to extend its meaning from that usage.

Now art, as we have before had occasion to remark, always retains its contact with sense. In this respect it is different from other forms of experience that are often associated with it or compared with it. It is different from religion. For, though religion may often, perhaps must often, be sensuous in character, it does not seem necessary that the religious experience should always, or at every point, retain its adhesion to the sensuous. It seems, in fact, an essential of religion that it should, at some point, sever its connection with outward things, and strive, as far as possible, after an experience that is non-sensible and non-sensuous. Would it be unfair to find in the universally sensuous quality of art its *differentia* from religion ? In so far as art is vitally and continuously attached to sense, I do not think that it would.

Again, art contrasts with thought in as much as the latter, also, like religion, seems to be characterised— again, not necessarily or always, yet at certain points —by a severance from outward things. The mention of this fact need not be taken as raising the question whether eventually art or thought can furnish the profounder form of experience. In any case, however profound the experience given through art may be, it can never be of such a kind as to take us away from sensation. Sensation, or the sensuous, may be regarded, as on one side, the goal of art.

ART AND THE UNCONSCIOUS

By contrast with thought or with religion, we cannot afford to dispense with consideration of this fact of the ultimate sensuous character of art. That is to say, there is one aspect of art through which the orientation involved in its creation, or in its enjoyment, must always be outward, and outward in the most literal sense. It involves contact with something in space. For enjoyment of beauty, one must see or hear, or experience some kind of sensuousness. This means that whatever account we are to give of the inward movement in art, or of the inwardly directed orientation of the artist, it must be in harmony with the fact of the continual presence of sensation throughout the experience. In art, too, we are most especially concerned with sensations of sight and hearing—sensations which, in their very nature, are always of things lying at a distance beyond the periphery of the body.

It is conceivable, then, that the inward movement or moment discernible in the artist's orientation will not be exactly the inverse, or exactly the antithesis, of the outward. At all events, and whatever mode of expression we may use, we must beware of trying to render our task too easy by the mere facile supposition that the outward moment in art will be explained just by asserting about it the contrary of what might have been said of the inward ; or just by conceiving it as a movement in a diametrically opposite direction. For, it must be remembered, while our initial point of view gave us a certain positive conception of the representative in art as arising through the artist's absorption in outward things—literally outward, out there in ' real ' space—when we tried to envisage the problem of form, we had to begin merely in a negation. We conceived that it was in the shutting out or the obscuring of the object in space that the formal qualities of the picture or the statue began to emerge. The difficulty is, therefore, on a parallel with the one

154

involved in the antithesis of outer to inner. We can easily give a positive and literal meaning to 'outer;' but we can only find the significance of ' inner ' through the negative conception that it is what arises in experience when the ordinary avenues of sense are closed.

The true significance, in fact, of the idea of inwardness only appears when we can lift it out of its spatial implications.

The question is, then, can we by starting with a negative conception of form as that phase or moment which tends to obscure the outer object, eventually discover a more positive definition ? I ask the question, not so much in the hope of being able to furnish an answer, as to make it clear that, whatever answer might in the last resort be given, it cannot be found merely by supplying ourselves with opposites or contraries to the ideas of representation.

Once again, if we take West and East as symbolical of the outward and the inward, it need not be in the last resort that we should find them purely antithetical or contrary. We might begin by saying that the Eastern genius is given by the negation of Western activity, but we should at least admit that the last word had not been said. The Eastern genius must surely be capable of some positive mode of description. Finally, the difference between East and West has been taken to express or reflect an issue that captures the highest interests of the whole human race. If, therefore, we should link up our discussion of the formal or rhythmic problem in art with the problem of the values of the East and of the West, it would indicate our intention in two respects : first, that of trying to discover a positive—and not merely negative —significance in the idea of form and rhythm ; and second, of implying that the whole problem is worth while, because it is one of the great, real problems of philosophy.

(2)

With the larger significance in view, or in the hopes eventually of disclosing to ourselves the vaster issue, let us begin with the narrower meanings. There is an outward—a spatially outward ; and there is an inward—an inward that is defined, at all events, by the negation of the outward.

The artist, then, may be conceived as working through two possible orientations. He may keep his attention upon the object and strive simply in the plasticity of his medium, to see it afresh or have the new artistic vision of it. Or, on the other hand, with diminishing or vanishing attention to the object, he may strive to mould the medium according to its own nature, or its own laws. In so far as the first orientation requires a concentration of attention on the object, it will exclude the second. In so far as the second arises through withdrawal of the attention from the object, it will exclude the first. Now, I fancy that in the whole wide range of the world of art, we should have all degrees of this mutual exclusion. In some cases, for a very long time the artist's attention may be concentrated on the object ; and the form which is nevertheless emerging more and more all the time, receives no share of his attention. In other cases, conceivably, there will be rapid alternations between absorption in the object and withdrawal of attention from the object. In still other cases, the attention may be rarely directed to the object and the second kind of orientation will prevail, over the greater part of the time. Then, perhaps, there will be those cases where alternation of orientation is so rapid that they will be difficult to analyse ; or finally those cases where the difference between the two orientations is so slight, that the movement of alternation eludes any kind of observation. There might, indeed, be that case where the artist is able to keep the two antithetical aspects of the process within a single span of his attention. I think, however, that this is to be regarded as a limiting case —one that expresses the moment of balance between the two orientations when the transition from the one to the other is slow. I do not think it represents a sufficiently stable attitude for long-continued or effective work ; or that it is an attitude really typical of artistic intuition.

Up to this point we have been handicapped through our necessarily negative mode of defining the second orientation. We have always had to define it through the turning away of attention from the object. It would be natural, therefore, when we are now in search of some more positive means of definition, to ask whether the medium itself may not become, shall we say ? the secondary object of attention. In the orientation of the artist in which he withdraws himself from the object, does he not let his attention focus upon the medium itself ? I agree that it is worth while to ask this question ; but I should anticipate later conclusions by pointing out that, were we to abide finally in such a view, it would negate the essential function that, more and more, we have been attributing to the medium. For a medium is that which mediates, and if the clay become an object of attention in and for itself, so far forth must it be felt to renounce its mediatory function.

There is, however, a very great deal in human sensibility, in the testimony of artists themselves, and in the critical investigation of the nature of art, that, as it were, cannot help pausing to enjoy the delightfulness of the material thing that pleases the eye or that responds to touch and pressure with its mere crystalline fabric, or its golden heavy malleability. It almost seems as if there were a moment in the whole artistic process in which the artist does concentrate his attention on the medium. It is almost as if the sheer delightfulness of the material were a kind of by-path meadow—as if it offered an irresistible temptation to wander about in aimless enjoyment.[1] There is here, I think, at once a real value and a real danger. It is the fascination of the medium—its particular kind of plasticity—that calls his attention away from the object ; and we may conceive this as absolutely necessary, otherwise he would be lost in absorption in the object. It is also, however, as if the mere seductive power of the medium offered no positive cue towards the further definition and limitation of his attention. Thus when art loses itself in the effort to exhibit the richness of gold or ivory, or the strangeness or novelty of orchestral tones, it becomes at once debased. Granting then, that it is legitimate and necessary to enter for a moment upon the luxuriance of by-path meadow, how is the artist, so to speak, by a loop line, to find his way back to the king's highway ? He may scarcely evade the temptation of its seduction ; yet how is he, as it were, to overcome the medium, and to get beyond it, while yet retaining its values of mediation ; to secure his goal and keep its fascination in subservience to an intention which is his very own ?

Let the artist's attention be supposed to come to rest, for a moment, in the medium. This arresting of the attention by the medium, this playing of the interest round the medium, is beautifully elucidated and interpreted at all events from the point of view of critical appreciation, by Bosanquet in his *Three Lectures on Æsthetic.* I mean, that this is Bosanquet's own attitude in these lectures. He has caught the very living spirit of that phase in artistic experience

[1] Note to what extent modern music has fallen a victim to this temptation.

where the medium arrests alike the mind and the sensibility ; and it is the flickering of the attention round and round the medium and upon different varieties of media that constitutes the elusiveness and the charm of the book. By an amazing felicity of illustration, he makes Homer his spokesman, he catches Homer at the very instant when the poet's attention was arrested by the gold of which the shield of Achilles was made. " It is," the philosopher remarks of his illustration, " perhaps the earliest æsthetic judgment which Western literature contains. It is in the Homeric description of the metal-working deity's craftsmanship in the shield of Achilles. He has made upon it the representation of a deep fallow field with the ploughmen driving their furrows in it ; and the poet observes, ' And behind the plough the earth went black, and looked like ploughed ground, though it was made of gold ; that was a very miracle of his craft.'

" Now what was the miracle here, that made Homer cry out at it with delight ? It was not, surely, that when you have one bit of ploughed land you can make another like it. . . . Surely the miracle lies in what Homer accents when he says, ' Though it was made of gold.' "

" *Though* it was made of gold." It is the emphasis upon the " though " that expresses the spirit of Bosanquet's thinking in these lectures and makes him so charming—and so elusive. For he is very elusive. It is as if the arresting of his attention by the metallic gold challenged him to the battle with it. He is at once eagerly, ardently appreciative of the value of gold ; and yet he always seems to think of it as something that had to be deprecated.

Now, there seems to me no eventual access to the problem of art, unless we can change this ' though ' into a ' because.' The miracle must ultimately be found to lie *in virtue of* the thing's being made of gold. For so long as we retain the negative conjunction, we shall never find the way towards a positive insight into the formal character of art ; and so Bosanquet is never able to give any indication of the way. Deeply as he is impressed with the power of those arts, whose essence it is to be formal, he can only envisage that power through the negation of the representative. A little further on we find the sentence : " Yet the idea for example that in music we have the pure type of expressiveness, that towards which every art is bound o aspire, does appear to indicate an inherent impulse of the art-spirit towards a mode of utterance which is not loaded with the weight of representation." " Which is not loaded with the weight of representation." Further than that negative he does not take us.

In that exclamation of Homer's, there is certainly an implication in the ' though.' There is, apparently a disadvantage in the shield's being made of gold. It prevents it from being quite like the ploughed field; but just because it is not like the ploughed field, it must have some other appearance, it must be even *like* something else ; it must send the mind or the sensibility off in some other direction and away from the ploughed field. Now, as we have seen, it might send the mind off in the mere enjoyment of the gold ; but if it does not do more than that, we should not have the really beautiful thing that aroused the Homeric wonder.

The problem then is to find the positive principle operating within this new orientation of the mind forced upon it, initially, by the gold.

Could we not take our cue, once more, from the chance (?) occurrence of the word, Western, in Bosanquet's illustration. It would be natural for the Western poet to go instinctively to the representative value of the workmanship, and therefore to say ' *though* ' it was made of gold. As opposing this

instinct, we might place the movement of contemporary art criticism and evaluation that leads towards
the art of the East, and the recognition of its peculiar
values, and that lays so great stress upon the formal
side of painting. The East, it is said, with its relative
indifference both to outward things and to the science
which relates them and governs them, can show an
art of far greater formal power. Is not this, indeed,
the true orientation of all painting towards form—not
towards representation ?

Here, however, it is possible to reach a too hasty
conclusion. Some critics have, it is true, gone wisely
to Eastern art, and with a profound sense of its inner
differences from that of the West. Such minds as
Mr. Lawrence Binyon have perceived, and emphasised,
the danger that would threaten the art of both, should
either be tempted uncritically to adopt the other's
values. Other critics, like Mr. Roger Fry and Mr.
Clive Bell, with less insight into the divergence of
mentality between ourselves and the East, have supposed that because the East can show power over form
that the West cannot show, therefore, the values
of all painting lie essentially in formal qualities.

Have they, in working out their view of form,
given us a really adequate account of it ? For they
incline to speak of it as something that can be achieved
independently of representation ; or at the least, they
produce upon the reader's mind an impression of
tearing it asunder from the representative effects
which are its vehicles. Analysis of their view will, I
think, serve to elucidate the immediate issue.

Mr. Roger Fry in emphasising the importance of
form in the æsthetic evaluation of a picture instances
The Transfiguration of Raphael, and shows, con-
vincingly so far as part of his argument goes, that the
disposition of the masses of colour is an all-important
factor in the æsthetic impression—' the spatial

relations of plastic volumes.' He speaks, however, of the ' dramatic insincerity ' of the picture, indicating thereby that its æsthetic value must be found along lines that diverge from its representative effect. He calls the figures at the foot of the mount " academic gentlemen in impossible garments and purely theatrical poses." The æsthetic unity of the picture must therefore be found in spite of this dramatic insincerity. What, then, is its vehicle ?

Can the significance of the book—the ' plastic volume '—with which a scribe—the ' academic gentleman '—is preoccupied at the foot of the mountain be a *merely* formal one ? It must, of course, *be* a formal one ; but can it be that alone ? The impression produced through the position, shape and colour of such a mass relative to other masses, is conditioned by the impression that the mass itself makes upon the eye. That is to say, it has the representative effect of being understood as a book. Now a book in relation to masses of colour has a different æsthetic effect from some other white surface. Formal relation is conditioned by the representative effect of the term of the relation.

It is scarcely true, then, as Mr. Fry seems to indicate, that the scribe's preoccupation with the book is altogether to be put down to dramatic insincerity, or is altogether out of harmony with the vastness of the subject. A book is as significant as the transfiguration itself. A book is the storm-centre of the universe. That is why Raphael makes his scribe point to a book. While it is true, therefore, that there is a unique majesty of rhythm in the relative position of the white page to other parts of the picture, that peculiar relation is effected only because the white page is a page—of a book.

This means that formal power is gained by employing representative effect. In a picture, however, there must be an eventual subservience of form to representation.

There is, in fact, no greater wisdom in saying that the goal of painting is to produce " significant form "[1] than in saying that the goal of music or architecture is to produce representative effect. This indeed would be the opposite, and correlative, error. Let us try to illustrate it. Consider the inexpressibly austere beauty of the triforium of Notre Dame. Supposing someone wished to maintain the view that apparently formal arts like architecture and music could be beautiful only in virtue of the subtle representations involved in their rhythms ; that would be the paradox, for these arts, correlative to Mr. Fry's for the art of painting. In order to do so, such a theorist would have to say that the triforium of Notre Dame was beautiful because it is like the majesty one sees only upon the face of the dead. So it is. That amazing repose and aloofness of the threefold rhythm of the arches *is* like " the fixed evanescence "[2] in the countenance of death. Yet that resemblance is part only of the whole experience, a secondary part, too, and one that must be absorbed in the more dominant aspect of its totality, the rhythmic aspect, if that experience is to reach its goal. Just as, in the picture of Raphael, the formal quality of the relations of the masses is conditioned by, and absorbed in, the representative quality of the whole; so, in the contemplation of the triforium of the cathedral, the subtle and elusive resemblance, conditioned by the rhythm, is also absorbed by it and essentially subservient to it. In neither case may the orientation appropriate to each work of art be entirely lost. In the first case, the picture must be thought, felt and apprehended as a picture of something. In the second case, the architectural design must be thought, felt and appre-

[1] *Art.* Clive Bell.   [2] George Macdonald.

hended as something that in its very nature precludes the direct representation of any real object.

The contrast between Notre Dame and the picture of Raphael is very marked. They typify entirely different species of art, and show the differentiation between the representative tendency and the rhythmic carried to a high degree. It is clear that whatever representative effects or suggestiveness is discernible in the rhythms of the triforium of Notre Dame must fall entirely within the rhythmic and become absolutely subservient to rhythm ; and it is equally clear that whatever formal power the picture of Raphael may possess must become wholly subservient to what we have called the outward or objective orientation of the painter. I am not disinclined to the view that this is one of the excellencies of the Western art spirit —the severity, the precipitate and uncompromising character of its specific differentiation. It will have yea or nay. It will make *either* form *or* representative effect its goal, or its governing value. So that, in European art as a whole, we find the extreme of Renaissance representative technique on the one hand, and the extreme of pure formal instrumental music on the other.

But it is not so in the East. There it is far harder to discern the watershed between the flow of the art spirit towards the goal of decoration and formal design, and the movement of it that leads to picture painting as such, or that can be thought as painting through the analogy of the Western art. Hence even where the Eastern spirit is most unmistakeably decorative and formal in aim, it achieves this intention through an enormously greater variety of representative forms ; while in its painting where the decorative intention is kept in subordination, it is nevertheless in subordination to a far less degree than in the West. That is why it pleases the school of Western criticism that is so ardent in its search for ' pure ' form. Here undoubtedly are to be found the peculiar art-values of the East, but Mr. Binyon's warning expresses exactly the danger that lies in a too hasty attempt towards their appropriation. " Ignorant," he remarks, " of all that lay behind these strange, new, ravishing harmonies of line and colour, enthusiasts were prompted to imagine that here at last was an ideal art, produced by men who were concerned solely with problems of decorative- design, indifferent to subject. And under this spell are those in Europe who imagine that our artists should do likewise."[1]

Eastern decorative art is the term we need in order to exhibit that phase of the artist's orientation now under consideration. Here the decorative artist is employing a variety of representative effects, as it were, to scatter or disperse the attention—to diminish the absorption of the mind in any one object by presenting a variety of other objects along with it. Now if that variety of objects tended to bring back the attention to the original central object, we should have, so far, only the outward orientation of the painter ; but in so far as the variety is presented in order to lead the mind away from any central object, we have the tendency towards the orientation that negates absorption in the outer world, towards the orientation that is, by contrast, inward in character.

Suppose, next, the variety of objects that radiate out from, rather than converge towards, anything like a centre of interest, are themselves presented with a high degree of symmetry or rhythmical arrangement. This, I fancy, could be well illustrated from Venetian decorative architecture, which, indeed, might be taken as an approximation to a link between East and West. At all events, we have something that comes very close, now, to the merely formal arrangement of

[1] *Painting in the Far East*, p. 254.

M

architectural elements in a purely architectural and non-representative design. Suppose, therefore, that we take the last step, and negate, as completely as possible, any representative effect in the several elements that constitute the symmetry or the rhythm. We arrive at architecture—architecture of the West, with the pure severity and concentration of its mass effects—that of which we have taken the triforium of Notre Dame as our type, but of which either Greek or Romanesque architecture is still more purely typical.

It is, at this point, I think, in so far as the arts of the visible and the visual are concerned—those arts that either lead the mind outward to space, or in which the finished artefacts are themselves planted in space, and whose impressiveness involves spatial implications that may be both vast and definite—that we arrive at the most complete negation of representative effect— the rhythm of architectural elements. Can we pass directly from this spatial rhythm to the temporal rhythm of music ? It is in this transition, if it can be effected, that I should look for the positive quality of rhythm as opposed to its definition through the mere negation of representative effect. It is the transition from rest to motion, which, with all the implications that it has for art, raises the new and tremendous question of emotion. All art is emotional ; and every kind of art has its own peculiar kind of emotion. Music is movement, literally, and in a sense that no sculpture, painting or architecture ever could bear. Its emotion is such an obvious feature of it, and its movement comes with such a manifest impressiveness, that the relation of the word, emotion, to the word, motion, ceases here altogether to be one of mere metaphor or analogy. The motion and the emotion of music must surely be integrally and articulately related.

We have hitherto been regarding rhythm and form as alternative expressions for the same fundamental idea. Let us now separate them and try to analyse the implications of each term. Rhythm implies movement in a way that form does not. Rhythm is primarily and naturally applied to a temporal sequence, and only by a kind of courtesy to the spatial dispositions of a picture or a building. Now especially in architecture, the idea of form implies the idea of energy. Schopenhauer, with that mingling of insight and felicity of exposition which is his peculiar genius, shows how essential it is that the formal lines of architecture and the formal relations of the masses of a building should express, for the sensibility, the gravitational forces in virtue of which the building coheres and has unity as a building. In architectural form, therefore, there is implied the idea of energy. The masses of the building, though at rest, stand to each other in a relation that can be interpreted only through the idea of potential energy, and that the sensibility in its own way must thus interpret.

Even in a picture, the opposition of mass to mass involved in its formal harmony, produces a parallel effect upon the sensibility. There is the same sense, though less characteristically, in painting, of potential energy in the distribution of line and colour.

Returning to rhythm, in its simple application to a temporal series, it is quite easy to find in it an expression of kinetic energy. It is easy even in poetry. In music, it is one of the most striking things about that art.

With the impression of movement and energy implied in rhythm and form there is involved the emotional effect that belongs to all art ; but it is revealed more clearly in the rhythm of music. Music is movement in a literal sense—literal, at least, in so far as it means progression in time. If we pass into art that is always in immediate conjunction with music—dancing—we have also movement in space. Even, however, limiting ourselves to music, we begin to perceive how this transition from spatial form to temporal rhythm must force the emotional aspect of art upon our attention.

I think, then, that the main initial conception from which we ought to work is the emotional character of music. At first sight, it may look arbitrary, or at the least, raise a challenge, when one attempts to relate the idea of emotion in art specifically to form and rhythm. Music, however (with dancing) is without exception or reservation that art in which rhythm, in the narrowest sense of the term, is predominant ; and prevails to an extent which leaves even poetry far behind. Of course, rhythm is *essential* to poetry ; but poetry is not ' made of ' rhythm in the sense in which music is made of it.

And music is the most emotional of the arts. It is that art which carries, or may carry, emotion to the highest degree of intensity. It is often called an art of feeling ; and all our sensibility ascribes to music an emotional lordship over the other arts. I should point, therefore, to the relation between the tremendous emphasis of beat or accent in music and the primitive emotional effect that such accentual rhythm has upon our sensibility as affording us a principle that we could apply in less obvious cases. Dancing is almost on the same plane, but dancing is hardly ever, if at all, dissociated from music.

On the other hand, those arts where temporal rhythm is impossible, bring emotions of an altogether austerer type. Painting or sculpture never produce the Dionysiac effects of music. Their proper emotions are altogether different. Pure drama, without music, holds a kind of middle position. With its temporal rhythms, both of verse, and of dramatic sequence, it can produce emotions of relatively high intensity. When it goes in the direction of the highest intensity, it enlists the aid of the ballet, or passes into music drama. The finest pure dramatic emotions, those that belong to dramatic situations as such, or to the rôle of the chorus in the Greek stage, tend to a certain austerity within which music does not need to limit itself.

It is, I think, important to stress the emotional austerity of the two representative arts, painting and sculpture, that are precluded in their nature from expressing anything in a temporal sequence. They are arts that involve the direction of the artist's attention upon the outer world, while at the same time they have this limitation—which poetry has not —of not being able to present any kind of temporal rhythm.

Now why is it that the arts of representation should tend towards austerity of emotion and that the arts of form and rhythm—and especially those of temporal rhythm—should tend towards intensity of emotion ? ' Austerity ' and ' intensity ' are perhaps not adequate expressions of the two diverse qualities, but they may serve as indications. At all events, it is in the answer to this question, or to a question something like this, that I should attempt to find the means of changing our hitherto negative view of the artist's inward orientation into a positive definition of his aim.

Especially with reference to music, the word, mood, and the idea of the expression of a mood, are significant and important. With more point than in the case of painting, the musician who sits down to the piano-forte to improvise may be said to have in view the expression of a mood. There might be some justification, then, for taking the emotion of the artist as the thing that, in music, initiates the artistic process and indicates or defines its general direction. Whereas for the painter the initiatory exclamation might be, " Oh ! I must draw that mountain ! " for the musician it would rather be, " I feel sorrowful, I must play." In the first case, the accent is upon the object—the mountain. In the second case, the accent is upon the emotion, but not so much as an object as an experience. In the first case the object is ' out there,' and has the permanence and the repose of things that some kinds of painting, at all events, take delight in contemplating. In the second case, the emotion, as experience, is drawn out in time, and easily expresses itself in a way that marks its temporal character. Nothing could do this better than rhythm, in the narrow sense.

(4)

The antithesis between the two orientations, then, has condensed into something like the difference between absorption in an object of outer nature and the search for experience. Even so, the idea of ' search for experience ' remains sufficiently nebulous by contrast with the idea of vision directed upon the natural landscape or the human form. Since the experience is necessarily in the future and so far forth on the lap of the gods, to speak of the search for it may perhaps recall the ecstasy of the nigger at the revival meeting—" I'se gwine ter have a 'sperience " —without affording any more light than he is able to give as to the actual character of the 'sperience when it shall be forthcoming. Since, however, the problem of giving definition to the impending experience has puzzled many wiser—or if not really wiser, at least more subtle—heads than his, the initial indefiniteness of his approach to experience may perhaps be forgiven him.

For very many, if not all, of the greater artists seem to have approached their work in such bewildered indefiniteness. Goethe, of course, has given a classical account of this mood of perplexity—the perturbed and obscure emotions, the void and formless unrest that *may*, if strongly dealt with, issue in the clear and victorious forms of art. But for Goethe the problem was always to be solved—and in the very nature of the case—only by turning to the outer world of men and women, of real friendship and of real love. With the musician it *cannot* so be solved, and it is in the nature of the case that it admits of no such solution. Love and friendship are, of course, necessary conditions ; but should his attention, like the poet's, become wholly absorbed in these outward things he will be no perfect or representative exponent of his art. For that art requires an eventual concentration upon the mood itself.

How is this concentration to be achieved ? My answer is that it must be in the discovery of some means through which a more perfect correlation can be found between mood and medium. Now this correlation involves the attribution of a relatively higher importance to the medium than in the case of the arts of outward orientation. Just because ' mood ' offers relatively so vague and difficult an object for the focus of the artist's concentration, the medium must be raised to a higher level of objective consideration ; and yet, in order that the medium shall not be divested of its true mediatory value, the musician may not lose himself wholly in it. He may do so only to the extent of helping his concentration towards the mood, and of not letting his attention fall too far outwards to the object.

Let us compare, for a moment, the musician in this respect, with the poet.

For both, emotion is of ultimate and supreme importance. Both may have the emotion, say, of sorrow, and the sorrow must reappear with the peculiar transfiguration that art can effect in the finished work of both. But the poet may allow his sorrow to express itself through the sorrow of other men and women. He can look out upon the world and ' see ' them sorrowful without knowing that it is his own sorrow that he sees in them. He can afford to cast his emotion forth, like bread upon the waters, even unknown to himself, and let it return to him through his ' vision ' of humanity. The musician cannot do this and does not do it. His emotion must be his own emotion, his very own, and as such it must find its æsthetic expression. His emotion is not to be lost or hidden in the object.

Consider for a moment, impartially, two such works of art as Bach's *Chaconne* and the first part of Goethe's *Faust*. Supposing Arnold were right in claiming for those passages in the latter which relate to Margaret an unsurpassable poignancy of sorrow, what a *profound* difference there is from the musician's in the means through which the sorrow is expressed ! The grief, the woe, is *out there*—in Margaret, between Margaret and Faust. Or, keeping to Bach's *Chaconne* as a kind of central point of reference, the perfect type of the musician's art, compare it with those utterances that express Dante's relation to Francesca, or Shakespeare's to Constance, or Ophelia, or Desdemona. In contrast to the emotion of these poets constituted through their relation to *other* human hearts, the musician's attitude is the arrogance and the challenge of the prophet—" Behold and see if there is any sorrow like unto *my* sorrow." *My* experience—essentially, and in full consciousness, mine.

The musician, then, must keep the emotion as his own and apprehend it as his own. Therefore he will, as far as possible, keep it rhythmical. He will choose, for its expression, the medium which is *par excellence* rhythm ; and thereby he will, partially at all events, exclude the outer objects which might absorb his emotion into themselves. Yet since the sensuous is continuously present in all art, since without sensation we do not have art, the medium must give this sensation while at the same time excluding, or tending to exclude, the objective implications which as a general rule attach to the sensible. It may even give intense sensations ; for music may be loud, and very loud. Here, indeed, it shows an intensive quality that I scarcely think can be parallelled in art.

We have seen, however, that it is not possible to say ' rhythm ' without saying also ' representation through rhythm.' There is no such lofty convention in art that does not also in some degree, however imperceptible, imply a reference beyond itself. For the musician, then, every rhythm means something other than itself ; it means the ride of the Valkyries, or the slow monotonous recurrence of the waves, or the trampling of the feet of the hosts that bear the dead. Even Bach's *Chaconne* is dance music, and, though in an almost infinite remoteness, there appear somewhere the forms of the dancers, intangibly vague.

Still, the outer object, though always there, does, in music, tend to recede ; and in certain cases, like the *Chaconne*, recedes indefinitely far. Music, therefore, offers an extraordinary suitability towards the inward orientation of art. The mood, with its temporal character of successive phases, and of weaker and stronger emotional accents, easily finds reflection in the temporal rhythm of musical sounds and its necessary alternation of weaker and stronger beats ; it passes into the sound and becomes identified with it. The sound—the sensation—is taken up into the mood and incorporated within it, thus depriving, or tending to deprive, the sensation of objective implication and reference. So again, I should repeat a remark made at an earlier stage—that music is, of all forms of experience, that which most nearly approaches the limit of being experience in and for itself, and not *of* objects otherwise distinguishable from the experience.

If this be so, or in so far as this peculiar kind of limit is reached, it becomes correspondingly difficult to distinguish the various terms through which we have so far tried to find access to the nature of art. Thus, the sensations that are taken up and incorporated within the musical experience do not convey, or imply, the externality of objects ; they do not even convey or imply the externality of the medium itself. The three main terms with which all along we have been concerned, viz., the experiencing subject, the medium and the object—in some sense, external— that lies beyond, thus lose their boundary lines and flow into each other. Or *tend* to flow into each other. For, of course, no limit as such is actually reached. Momentarily, the emotion experience which is music may, at its most intense, yield an utter loss of all sense of objectivity, but only for a moment. On the whole, there will be ebb and flow ; and the highest emotional tide will, in general, stop short of giving that complete loss either of the sense of the object or the sense of the subject towards which music always tends, but only tends. So that the boundary lines of the distinctions are never wholly washed away.

We shall still continue, therefore, to speak as if we could distinguish between the experiencing artist and the object of outer nature which stands over against him ; and as if within that distinction there fell also the medium and such part or aspect of the artist's own experience—the mood or the emotion— upon which it is conceivable that his attention is, in some sense, directed. Let us call, for simplicity's sake, the two possible foci of his attention, the outer object and the subjective emotion. Both foci are discernible, or are illuminated, in every kind of artistic experience ; but according to the relative increased brightness or intensity of illumination of the outer or the inner, we have the orientation characteristic of painting, etc., on the one hand, and of music, etc., on the other. Can there be those limiting cases in which the illumination discernible in each focus is of equal intensity ? Again, I raise the question ; but again, I incline to answer it in the negative, except in so far as it shows a transitional and unstable phase of a more specific and stable orientation. This quasi-mathematical way of generalising the problem would, however, have the advantage of giving us, so to speak, a perfectly general equation that, by change only of the constants, would be applicable to every kind of art, or to every aspect of the whole artistic process.

The method has this further advantage. It throws out the suggestion that, in certain cases, the two foci might coincide. What does this mean ? When one uses language typified in such a formula as ' projection of unconscious contents upon an object,' it may at first sight be hard to discern what the direction of the artist's attention really is. For, if the artist project upon the object an exceedingly rich ' unconscious ' content, and if this content also involve the emotions, would that not amount to the direction of his attention upon his own inward and emotional experience ? On reflection, however, the answer must be definitely, No. In so far as he ' sees ' that content, however rich, and in however emotional a fashion, as belonging to the object, his orientation has all the qualities and values of the outwardly directed kind. It may very well be, however, so far as the argument goes, that there may arise those cases in which the artist does not know, does not feel, does not in any wise apprehend, whether he 'sees' these things in the object or attends to them as experienced within himself. If those cases should be real, then they would be represented by the moving together or the coinciding of the two foci. Again, however, I have to ask : Are they real ? and again I am disinclined to admit that they are, except as limiting cases or transitional phases. Again, I should support the view that the security of touch, the mastery of the conditions of his problem manifested by the artist in his crowning achievements, always come by his being able, in the last resort, effectively to differentiate his orientation, as, on the whole, outward, or on the whole, inward.

And this brings out a point of great importance and significance. It matters, and it perhaps matters supremely, in what way the artist is able to differentiate his emotion for the purposes of his art and *qua* a genuine æsthetic emotion. It matters whether the apparent source of that emotion be in the object, in what he projects into the object and what he 'sees' in it ; or whether that source appear as his own experience—or, at least, *as* experience and not as object.

We are thus enabled to give more definite meanings to what has been before broadly indicated or symbolised by austerity *versus* intensity. Whether or not the emotion of painting, and of which painting ought to be the best vehicle and exponent, is rightly called austere, it certainly ought to be felt as though it arose in and through the objective source to which the representative power of that art can give an effective access. On the other hand, it may not be entirely fitting to call the peculiar kind of emotion that is best brought to consciousness through music 'intense' as opposed to some other relative 'austerity.' The point at issue is, that musical emotion, at its best and most characteristic, is brought to consciousness through experience in its temporal aspect and not by leading mind or sensibility out towards the object. The proper vehicle of musical emotion is temporal rhythm. Generally speaking, therefore, there will be no confusion in masterly artistic work, as to whether its æsthetic emotion is presented as having its main source in the object, or in experience as such. It is far easier, of course, to define what is meant by 'experience as such' through appeal to music with its obvious temporal sequence of tone and accent ; but the case of architecture does not present any ambiguity. Even though the rhythm of the spatial elements of architecture recall, in an infinitely subtle way, things elsewhere visible in the natural world, and thereby produce the associated emotions and present them in æsthetic form, the dominant emotion of architecture is not, and ought not to be, traceable chiefly to such shadowy recollections. It ought to appear as flowing out of the peculiar mood that a building can so splendidly induce ; and of the contemplation that is essentially experience and that cannot find an ultimate or satisfying goal in any object, nameable as such, that lies beyond the building itself.

This, of course, is said subject to all the general reservations already made ; and subject to the fullest consideration of the finest oriental work, in cases which may be exceedingly hard to differentiate as decorative or as tending towards an intention that is, by contrast, like that of Western painting, rather than towards decoration or design. In other words, it is always well to keep in view the possibility that, even for purposes of emotion, the two foci may sometimes coincide. In Western art, I urge, they do so but rarely, perhaps not at all.

PART II

SYMBOLIC or 'ETERNAL'?

> Modern criticism is apt . . . . to dismiss all that concerns the dramatic presentation of the subject as literature or illustration, which is to be sharply distinguished from the qualities of design. But can this clear distinction be drawn in fact?
>
> ROGER FRY.

CHAPTER I

RAVENNA

In proportion as an artist is pure, he is opposed to all symbolism,
ROGER FRY

Hardly one of the works of literature which, by the consensus of
generation, are reckoned great, possesses this quality of æsthetic
perfection.   MIDDLETON MURRY

(1)

WE have all along attributed to the artist a certain
standpoint. We have spoken as if he looked at his
object, or as if he had a certain relation to his own
emotions. This relation to the self or to the object
has, further, been regarded as always conditioned by
an idea—'the idea of conscious life,' or 'of conscious
reflection.' It follows that appreciative response to a
given work of art is likewise conditioned. The
responsive mind is seeking 'a vision of the object,'
and tries to find it through the given work of art;
and in this search for vision through the given art,
the mind that searches must obviously be conditioned
in its search through its ideas. The ideas, however,
with which we come to a work of art are necessarily
different from those which originated it in the mind of
its creator.

We thus return to our initial point of view—the
'idea' of reflective consciousness, the selective
meditation of the poet. We have only to consider, in
addition, the selective meditation of the reader.
What is it that makes him go to one poet rather than
another ? What is it that makes him find in certain
passages in the poet of his choice, a conspicuous

beauty ? And we perceive that however closely he may be in unison with the mind of the author, he is bound to see the object at which that author is looking from a different standpoint. And he is bound to see as an individual equipped with different intellectual and spiritual resources. Here comes in the power of the idea. Just as there are minds better equipped for moulding the plastic medium that stands between them and their object ; so there are minds better equipped for formulating the idea within the power of which the artist so keeps his regard fixed upon his object, or it may rather be, within the power of which the appreciative recipient has the vision through the given work of the artist.

This scrutiny and exploration of the idea is the function of criticism ; or it is the region in which criticism can effectively move and in which it can effectively express apprehension of the vision. Whether we regard the artist as looking outward upon nature, or inward upon his own emotions, his concentration upon the outer or the inner must be achieved initially through some kind of consciousness. Only something thus expressible in terms of consciousness, in terms of the ' idea ' in its widest sense, could enable him to make that gesture of psychological command through which he interposes his medium between himself and his object, or through the magic of which he can divest his emotion of the sterility of its practical and non-artistic expression. We had spoken, however, of the ' dying of the idea ' within the vision ; or we had supposed that in the play the idea had to die, as idea, in order that the characters might live.

It is natural to ask : What happens to the poet's ideational consciousness after the play has been written and produced ? The testimony of the poets is unambiguously to the effect that they win a new consciousness.

Goethe bears a very convincing witness to the
change which takes place in the whole psyche of the
artist after he has given birth to his work. Even
then the poet is still *vis-à-vis* his work ; and therefore
he may become his own critic. He may formulate
his new ideas, and scrutinise the new consciousness
through which he approaches the old work. Since,
however, not every poet has the gift of formulating
ideas, it may very well be that some poets are bad
critics of their own work, and are not able to place
their readers in true perspective with regard to the
object of their vision. Very few poets have, in fact,
been able to do this as well as Goethe.

The man with the special gift for formulating ideas,
for defining the standpoint from which the vision of
the object can best be seen, is therefore in requisition
here. In virtue perhaps of this very gift, critical
rather than creative, his attitude *vis-à-vis* the work of
art can never be quite the same as that of it screator.
This will be eminently true when the children of a
later age are confronted with the art of an earlier.
They are in possession of ' ideas ' which in the nature
of the case their fathers could not have had. Yet they,
too, must experience the same thing as the original
creative artist. They must yield up their ' ideas ' to
the vision ; and these must, in some wise die, or be
absorbed in it.

The critical response to art must, however, be
different from the creative act. Since the ' ideas of
the conscious reflection ' of the critic must be largely
different from those of the creative artist, they will
conceivably be less wholly absorbed in the vision, or
less entirely drunk up by the characters of the play.
There will be, conceivably, a certain residuum of idea,
not unimportant for the critic in the formulation of
his impression of the work of art. This, perhaps,
would be the most general case.

Yet even granting that in cases of very profound critical appreciation, the absorption of the idea by the vision were to take place on as large a scale as in the creative mind, there must still remain what I have called the residuum of idea, if the critic were indeed able to exercise his critical function. That means that in every case, the critical mind as opposed to the creative, will always bring to bear upon the situation certain 'ideas' that cannot, in their very nature, wholly enter into or fuse with the vision. It is, I think, in virtue of this latter kind of 'idea,' that the art consciousness of different individuals, and of different ages of history, can be related.

Judge then of the importance of this kind of 'idea.' It could only be in virtue of such ideas that criticism could become a developed and differentiated *organon* of the mind. This is perhaps a differentiation that has not yet taken place to any extent in the history of our civilization. It seems as if it were a special function of the consciousness of our evolution and of our history that is only beginning to come into activity in our own day. Surely, among all our needs, there can be none more pressing than the development of this side of our historical consciousness.

(2)

It is clear that our formula, 'the idea of conscious reflection,' or 'the selective meditation of the artist,' is often satisfied through the profounder reflection of the religious consciousness. European literature, from Dante to Dostoevsky, can afford at least one or two *good* instances in which the poet's brooding over the mysteries of religion leads him straight forward, slowly or rapidly as the case may be, to the exercise of his creative genius. It is mere pedantry to defend this point.

It does not by any means follow that religion is always, or necessarily, the inspiration of art. Beaudelaire and Villon were very great artists ; and certainly there is at least a *prima facie* qualm to be overcome in conceiving their art, as inspired by the service of religion. It is, however, easier to defend the view that art is essentially religious in origin, and in the sources of its inspiration by reference to arts other than literature. And there is something important and significant in this fact. It is at least reasonable to urge that the beautiful mosaics of Ravenna, the art of Giotto and the Italian primitives, the music of Palestrina, and much post-Reformation music up to Beethoven, are very really and genuinely inspired through the Christian consciousness. It is not nearly so obvious, it is a much more difficult case to defend, that the dramatic work of Shakespeare is inspired through that consciousness.

In so far then as it may serve our purpose to see how religious ideas as represented, say, by the Christian λόγος, become transformed in European art, we need to restrict our scrutiny to certain more or less clearly defined types. With the exception of Dante, the typical artists are here not specifically men of letters, but painters or composers or workers in fresco or mosaic. Keeping within these limits, however, we are enabled to state with much greater clearness and ease, an issue that is of the highest significance in the relation of religion to art. Afterwards, we can again take up the cue afforded by the poets, and ask how literature as a product of the distinctive genius of Europe, demands a modification or re-statement of our general conclusions.

The problem at issue is this. Art always involves an unconscious content. Following, therefore, the line of thought in our discussion of the origin of the imagination, we should expect it to exhibit this content as a symbol, or in a form that may at any moment present itself as a symbol. May it not, then, also be the function of art to discover new symbolism, or to initiate new symbolic values ?

On the other hand, in so far as art appeared as a relation of outer and inner, as an achieved harmony between terms that had otherwise been inharmonious, there is, in virtue of this satisfaction and achievement, no need for symbolism. For the symbol is, *ex hypothesi*, that which arises through a state of conflict, and offers the cue towards the solution of the otherwise insoluble problem.

Art, that is to say, from our present position appears under two aspects. It appears first as symbolical, as a moment of discontent, as an effort towards transcendence of the given experience. But it appears as well, in the intense satisfaction we know as beauty, the experience within which we would most willingly abide, the harmony which we would most willingly retain—in short, as the very negation of the transcendent principle in experience.

Or, from the point of view of religion, we might ask : When art is genuinely in the service of religion, can its function really be to initiate new symbolism, since the religion which it seems to serve is already rich with its own symbolic content ? Is its function not rather simply to acquiesce in the given symbolism, to adorn the old, rather than to discover the new ?

Let is ask these questions with respect to one of the earliest significant expressions in art of the religion of Western Europe.

Byzantine architecture, from the fifth to the seventh centuries, with its peculiar employment of mosaic as a form of decoration integral to its architectural character, represents the period when Christianity was enjoying the peace of its first complete victory.

The religion had obtained a secure hold, but the security was quite recent.

The symbols that are so beautifully enshrined in the apses of its basilicas, maintained their ground, more or less in the form first given them there, for many centuries throughout the Christian Church. Yet these symbols are not in themselves new. All that these early workers in mosaic have done is to give them a certain definiteness and fixity of form. Yet in placing the imprint of their peculiar art upon these symbols, they have rendered them things of superb and abiding beauty. Limiting the field to Europe, we find an epitome of this early symbolic movement in art in the mosaics of Ravenna. San Vitale, Sant Apollinare Nuovo, Sant Apollinare in Classe, and the Ursian Battistero have each their own individual beauty of mosaic work; but one of the mosaics of Sant Apollinare in Classe furnishes us with an instance at once of such simplicity and of such beauty, that it will be best to limit illustration of our questions to it alone.

Above the apse of Sant Apollinare in Classe, the four evangelists are represented in a fashion which theological tradition had already rendered current coin, viz., as the eagle, the angel, the lion and the ox, They are seen upon a background of the clouds of heaven, wrought in pieces of stone of exquisite colour and gold. This is in the sixth century. As early as the close of the second century, Irenæus[1], for example, had begun to focus this tradition through the images of the lion, the calf, the man, and the winged creature. That is sufficient to show that the artist of this mosaic did not by any means originate the symbol. At the very most, he expressed his own individual feeling towards a symbol, the essential terms of which were already given. Yet so huge is the

---

[1] *Irenæus*, III., 11, 8.

gulf between any mere oral or written tradition and the incorporation of its ideas in a device of coloured and gilded stone, that it is only fair to ask whether it be not also in certain essential respects, the creation of a new symbol.

For it takes over, as it were, a minimum of traditional material and embodies this minimum of tradition in a superbly beautiful way. Now what is the significance in the apparently so simple process of endowing a few bare and abstract symbolical conceptions—and these, too, already familiar—with such a resplendent and permanent beauty ?

May we not say that here in this mosaic we find brought together several of the profoundest instincts we know in human nature, and brought together in such a way that they all find satisfaction ? The harmony of the purple and gold of these clouds seems to take you up into the infinite heavens. I think, here, we may safely accentuate this feeling of exaltation and remoteness. When the mosaic was first completed, and for the earliest worshippers in the building, it certainly could not have been less impressive for them, as a piece of colour harmony, than it is for us twelve hundred years later.

But what are the infinite heavens ? Are they not just the projection of the unfathomable depths within ?

One often hears statements to the effect that art only reaches its goal when it is able to see things human against the background of the universe ; the mortal things that touch the mind through the delicate, intense, sensibility of art do so only in the power of some kind of infinitude. We have to ask, however, what account can be given, psychologically, of this idea of infinity, or rather—and for the sensibility as opposed to the intellect—of this perception or impression of infinitude. It must be conceived to arise, surely, in proportion to the depth from which emotion or imagination or any other content of mind or soul can be evoked by the means at the disposal of art. The extent of the perception, or if the word be preferred—of the illusion, of infinitude is a measure of the depths of the unconscious which have been sounded and brought within the conscious harmony of the vision. Since what is 'seen' without, is in reality a projection of what has lain hidden within, the exaltation, the remoteness, the infinitude of the vision is conditioned and measured by the profundity of the levels that have been reached in 'the unconscious.' The more archetypal the character of what is evoked, the greater the chances towards the illusion of infinitude in the thing seen. I do not say that depth of unconsciousness will certainly give 'infinitude,' but only that 'infinitude' is at least conditioned by archetypal depth.

Somehow, then, these early Christian workers in mosaics have known how to touch the depth. If we cannot say how they have known, at least we can observe one or two aspects of the process by which they came to do it.

Along with the sense of height and depth with which this mosaic impresses, there is also a wonderful sense of repose—a repose which indeed characterises all the beautiful things in Ravenna. This sense of repose is unquestionably the echo or the reflection of a living religion, but one which has nevertheless gained its ground and is free, for the time being, from the restlessness of contention or even of the spirit of initiation. This sense, at once of repose and of conviction, is expressed again, though perhaps in a more homely way, in the Battistero. There, just where the walls begin to curve into the dome, in the spaces between the four evangelists, are four curious little tabernacles—always in mosaic. I suppose they are intended for the privacy of the evangelists, when they should choose to retire to them. But since they remain always unoccupied, they exercise a fascination and a hypnotism upon you as you stand there below them. Those delightful little tabernacles between the evangelists—at once so cosy and so mysterious—are vacant evermore in still, seductive invitation to you to come in and sit down and write a gospel.

(3)

It will be difficult, in fact, to escape the contrast between the repose of this early Byzantine art and the restlessness of the Gothic spirit and of the art that begins, say, about the time of Dante.

I think, therefore, that I have good grounds for the formulation of the questions : Is not this a type of art that does not so much initiate or prophesy as acquiesce and confirm ? And what, psychologically, is implied in this kind of beauty ?

Religions rise and have their day and pass away again. Does the historical religion of the West differ in this respect from any of them, or has it any claim to permanency more than the others ? Let the reader answer as the logic of his own mind compels him. His answer, one way or another, will scarcely affect the supposition that there are certain structures or certain tendencies in the human psyche which are of so unalterable a character as almost to merit the epithet eternal. There is an instinct, for example, for man to represent his strength under the form of an animal that for dateless ages has always stood in his experience as the strongest animal form he knew—the lion, the leviathan, the dragon. Such an instinct we may consider as more primeval and more permanent than the specific tendencies that animate, for the time being,

any of the transitory historical religions, or—for the
benefit of the reader intent upon eternal values !—the
religion that supervened upon the world at so late a
date in its history as Christianity. Such an instinct,
too, we may suppose, would always find expression in
form and colour. Or rather, from a more primeval
standpoint, the forms and colours associated with the
appearance of the animal form in question, or the forms
and colours through which it met the eye and made its
challenge to the security of the mind, would themselves
pass into the archetypal form and become an integral
part of it. Thus, the winged creature has, throughout
the evolution of man, been seen against the sky ; and
so man can never see the eagle in any of his visions save
as against the purple and the gold of heaven. Not
only the animal form itself, but the forms and colours
through which it appeared or in which it might be
visualised or dreamed would pass into the very
structure of mind and brain. Not only would they
pass into the structure of mind and brain, they would
also embody themselves in the structure of eye and
visual perception. Just as the eye is an organ of an
immemorial evolution, so are the visual and visualising
powers of the mind built up out of forms and colours
associated or blended through far too long æons of time
ever to become separable again. The forms and the
colours and the things seen are, so to speak, not three
terms, but one term. This trinity in unity has been
in process of formation long before the ancestors of
man had become man. It goes back to his animal, to
his reptilian—if you like, to his protoplasmic—pre-
existences. In such a sense, then, the instinct for man
to see and to visualise his strength under the archetypal
animal form is, for want of a better word, eternal.
Now the reflective concepts of the religious consciousness, old as they are in history, represent something
far more recent than such primeval archetypes ; and

however deeply they may be rooted in such archetypes, they have something in them of a novelty that cannot be in any obvious harmony with the deeper layers of his soul. Their very novelty and creativeness seems to involve man in a psychological moment that thrusts him aside from his archetypes, or that even seems to run athwart them. The creativeness of any of the transitory, or the later religions that mark the stepping stones of his pathway seems to involve such a moment not fully in harmony with his archetypal nature. Christianity is here an excellent example. " The cross," or " the evangelist " does not belong to primeval man in the sense that the lion belongs to him. The cross and the evangelist are not archetypes in the sense in which the lion and the eagle are such. If, therefore, in the course of his religious experience he were merely to draw pictures of the cross and of the evangelists he might be doing something of religious significance— perhaps of the profoundest religious significance—but he would nevertheless not be an artist and could not come thereby to the experience of beauty.

But now suppose a pathway opens up before him along which he can bring his religious intuitions of the cross or of the evangelists into harmony with these archetypes of 'more eternal' standing, these archetypes that confront him out of the unconscious in the form of the primeval animal and the primeval bird—then a marvellous change, a marvellous illumination supervenes within his consciousness. The evangelists assume the shapes of the lion and the eagle ; but they take on these shapes not merely as shapes, but in the implication of the form-relations and the colour-relations that, through the ages of evolution, have become integral to the very primeval animal shapes themselves. Then there is consciousness of beauty. Then there supervenes in human experience that still glowing splendour of the Byzantine mosaic that takes you, as you please to call it, into the infinite heavens or down into the unfathomable depths.

Is this expression, then, in beautiful form and colour of a symbolic idea necessarily a further development of the symbol itself, or is it to be taken as the achievement of a harmony and the winning of a spiritual satisfaction that are not symbolical, but different or divergent from the symbolic intention ?

I think that, without any reservation, we must find room for both values. For on the one hand, the churches of Ravenna were meant for worshippers ; and if we denude the mosaics in their apses of their dynamic and religious interest and attraction, if we fail to invest them with their symbolical power, we take art altogether out of its place in human life. We must conceive, in some very simple terms, that the early Christian worshippers wanted to know what the evangelists were like, and what significance that knowledge might have for their religion. In some such way, we are bound, I think, to conserve the power of symbolism in art. Yet this dynamic aspect of art must not be separated from that aspect through which it presents itself as achieved harmony. For it was not only those early worshippers who looked up into the quiet, awful repose of their apses and felt the profound beauty of their mosaics. We also feel that beauty. And yet for us ' the cross ' and ' the evangelists ' are perhaps no longer important. They do not seem to stand, now, on the pathway along which we seek our *Erlösung*. Why, then, is it that these mosaics should still seem beautiful to us ? Or, to free the question from all entanglement with the Christian controversy, why is it that we can go to the profoundest religious art of the East and find it beautiful, without ever having fully or deeply shared in the religious conceptions of the East ? This last suggestion, however, carries with it but a modicum of conviction. Though undoubtedly East and West can meet more easily and more completely in their art than in any other way, I am doubtful how far that interchange of æsthetic emotion does really go, apart from mutual comprehension along other lines of experience beside those of art.

Granting, however, that some religious sympathy and contact are necessary for the appreciation of the art of any age or race, we must finally keep in view also the non-symbolical value of art in virtue of which it is harmony and repose rather than motion or self-transcendence. And it is this aspect of art that is exhibited on the whole rather more than the former by the Byzantine period that we have been considering. By contrast with the art of the later middle ages, the Gothic period, for example, I think we shall be able to say that Ravenna is typical of that spirit in art which does acquiesce in the traditional symbolism rather than set itself the task of devising new.

(4)

The antithesis between the dynamic or symbolical or self-transcendent in art, on the one hand, and its aspect of repose or harmony on the other should, I think, be illustrated by reference to the principle that in experience of beauty there is always a certain union of the perceiving mind with the object it perceives as beautiful. In this union we have the aspect of harmony and repose—the satisfaction in æsthetic contemplation upon which Schopenhauer so continually insists. But then, after the first ecstatic tide of emotion has passed away, we are none the less able to recall and review our experience. I do not think it is possible to estimate the value of beauty in human experience without also taking into account the power to recall and to review. For, whereas in beauty as harmony, something is realised through æsthetic emotion, something may now become accessible to our consciousness that had otherwise remained unrealised.

Here, again, there comes in what I have called the residuum of unabsorbed idea characteristic of the responsive or critical mind rather than of the creative. I am not so much concerned to show how this ' idea ' comes about as to urge that, in one phase of the total experience at all events, it must always be there. It may be that it emerges rather after the moment of ecstasy or of the pure self-sufficiency of beauty has passed away. It may be that it is present in some form all the time. At all events, I should like to conclude this brief reference to the art of Ravenna by asserting that one cannot do final justice to art without taking into account not only its ecstasy or its self-sufficiency, but also its ideational or cultural import.

It is the exploration of this cultural import that is the function of criticism. It is here, at all events, that criticism has an indubitable sphere where its right of scrutiny and inquiry cannot be challenged. It is within this sphere that many minds can meet and effect a vital interchange of ideas ; and it is here that the fellowship of mind with mind *vis-à-vis* the work of art can be vitally established. It is by moving on from this standpoint, and in virtue of this sympathy that a real concensus of opinion may perhaps be gained. What is important is not so much an attempt at ' objective ' judgment or evaluation of a work of art, as a higher degree of psychological rapport between one appreciative mind and another. Thus the ' idea ' of reflection can be formed and brought to focus within the collective consciousness that is confronted with the work of art ; and thus the art-consciousness of one age can be brought into relation with that of a later time.

CHAPTER II

The Gothic Spirit

It is that strange disquietude of the Gothic spirit that is its greatness ; that restlessness of the dreaming mind . . .

RUSKIN

(1)

BETWEEN the majestic simplicity of Byzantine mosaic, which has been taken to represent the earliest articulate expression of Christianity in art, and the age of Dante and of Gothic architecture, there intervenes roughly a period of some five or six centuries. Now it is clear that in that lapse of time, and in view of the character of European history, profound changes must have supervened upon the earlier and more primitive religious consciousness. Yet Gothic architecture or the poetry of Dante or the art of Giotto are perfectly authentic utterances of the Christian Spirit. Limiting consideration to architecture alone, the Byzantine, the Romanesque and the Gothic are plainly expressions of a single religious attitude.

How, then, are we to interpret the obvious differences between, say, the two end terms of these—the Byzantine and the Gothic. Volumes have, of course, been written and could still be written on these differences in their detail. Is there, for our purpose, any way of bringing the complexity of the detail under a single point of view ?

The critical and appreciative tendencies of the present for the most part go out towards primitive art and towards those types of art which are severe, simple and that show a high degree of purity and perfection of form. This critical tendency is, I have no doubt, in deep psychological accord with the profounder spiritual requirements of our age. It stands in contrast, for example, to the Romanticism of last century and to the revival of interest in Gothic art. The twentieth century has manifested what almost amounts to a reaction against the Gothic revival.

But if we review with a little greater care some of the things that were said in praise of Gothic architecture during the epoch from which the children of our day are so much in revolt, we should find the older attitude towards Gothic not so much out of harmony with our own as might at first be supposed. I do not think more real justice was ever done to the Gothic spirit than by Ruskin in *The Stones of Venice*. It is, therefore, significant when we find that he denies to its architectural expression those very qualities of formal perfection the absence of which its present-day critics are so eager to emphasise. What wins the admiration of Ruskin as the main positive contribution of Gothic is its power of grotesque. Yet grotesque, somehow, is not to be brought wholly within the unity of architectural purpose that can give the purity of design belonging to the greatest architectural schools. Here is a quotation that brings out the point quite simply and clearly.

"There is very little architecture in the world which is, in the full sense of the words, good and noble. A few pieces of Italian, Gothic and Romanesque, a few scattered fragments of Gothic cathedrals, and perhaps two or three of Greek temples, are all that we possess approaching an ideal of perfection. All the rest—Egyptian, Norman, Arabian and most Gothic, and which is very noticeable, for the most part all the strongest and mightiest—depend for their

power on some development of the grotesque spirit."
The remarkable thing about this passage is that it
implies that "all the strongest and mightiest" Gothic
is somehow not perfectly "good and noble" art.
This is surely a paradox. Could we resolve it by
saying that it is at once true, and yet the greatest
compliment that could be paid to the Gothic spirit?

A Gothic cathedral like Chartres passes through
such an enormous range of experience; and if it fails
to comprehend that experience within a single span,
it is hardly matter either for regret or for reproach.
Yet, let us observe, it is impossible to say that the
expressiveness of Gothic falls apart into the separate
types of beauty of its different elements. If it be true
that the power of all the strongest and mightiest
Gothic depends on some development of the grotesque
spirit, it is true also that the grotesque belongs to the
outside of the cathedral. What is as significant for
the interior as grotesque for the exterior is the window
with its coloured glass; not the architectural beauty
of the aperture alone, nor the colour with which it is
filled, but both together. Now while it is obvious
that the architectural effect of grotesque cannot be
had through the same visual impression as the architectural effect of the stained glass window, the two
effects do not fall entirely apart as though of two
different works of art. They fall within the compass
of what is at least a single experience, even if it be not
one of perfect æsthetic unity.

It is Ruskin, again, I think, who points out the
difference between such a building as Chartres, whose
soul is in its windows and such an one as the Sistine
Chapel, whose soul is in its walls and roof. It seems
to me, however, that the Gothic building contrasts
in this respect *both* with the Sistine Chapel of the
sixteenth century and the basilica of the sixth. Just
as Michael Angelo puts his soul into the roof of the

former, so the mosaic worker puts his into the apse of the latter. For neither mind do the windows have any significance other than that of affording light for what is within.

In the great period of Gothic this is quite clearly not the sole function of the window. Here the window has a function of its own to perform that is not merely important but central within the architectural effect. The apse, for example, is not only a resting place for the eye which there finds the goal of its architectural satisfaction. The apse is characteristically filled with colour and becomes the focus, the point of maximum intensity, of the beauty of the whole.

Nowhere, perhaps, in the whole range of art, could we find an instance that would so exactly fit our old formula of " seeing an object through a medium," as the glass of the great period of Gothic architecture, say the twelfth century. In the case of the best glass of Chartres or Poitiers, or Bourges, less clearly and certainly, of Rouen or Canterbury, what you always ' see ' ultimately and finally, is the blue sky beyond, " the body of heaven in his clearness." The greater number of the windows of Chartres show this, most simply, perhaps, that of *Notre Dame de la belle verrière*. The window of the crucifixion in Poitiers shows it with a peculiar emotional intensity, and is perhaps the best illustration to be given of this quality of the Gothic spirit that I am trying to articulate. In the Christ the crucifixion in the lower part of the window, the cross is of ruby red, seen against the sapphire background of the sky ; but the aureole of the Christ is pale as of the colour of ashes, while the aureole of the risen Christ, above, is once more of sapphire blue—the aureole is the sky itself.

It is astonishing how soon, as regards stained glass, this ' transcendent ' spirit in the Gothic declines and palls—how soon the window becomes a mere picture and instead of being the point of transcendence allows the mind to rest content in the mere picture, or even hushes it, or subdues it, back into the cathedral. That most wonderful instinct manifested by the Gothic workmen to transcend the limits of his experience in grotesque or in stained glass has a very brief period of expression ; but it is this instinct of transcendence that is the very essence of Gothic.

It arises, clearly, from the greatness of the range of experience through which the workman is trying to pass and to the severity of the limitations placed upon him and within which he must work.

In grotesque, it is the expression of something new and challenging within him—a new attitude of his soul to the problem of evil. The grotesque is doubtless the earliest *artistic* formulation of the modern spirit of wit and laughter or of its germ. Almost contemporary with the great period of Gothic, we have in France what might be called the origins of *opéra comique*. But then, brilliant as the wit of these must have been, they are at this time pure improvisations. The grotesque of architecture, rudimentary, inarticulate, undifferentiated as it is in respect of the comic spirit, is nevertheless a formulation of that spirit that gains its immortality in one of the noblest types of European art.

The stained glass window represents the effort to transcend experience in another way. It would perhaps be simple, and not inaccurate, to epitomise this effort as the longing of Dante *riveder le stelle.*

The Gothic builders had behind them the experience of five or six centuries of the Christian era more than the workmen of Ravenna. That experience, momentous both on its outward and its inner side, left its due imprint upon the age. The epoch of early Christianity was primitive if in no other way than that it could not have had the experience of the age of Dante. With the advancing centuries life began to acquire a content that it was more difficult, but equally urgent, to express in art.

(2)

Dante's own problem was, in fact, too vast ever to admit any facile solution—to admit of any solution that can be brought under the formula of an æsthetic perfection.

For his problem was that of keeping together, in intuitive vision and sensibility, as well as in knowledge, worlds so different, and so opposed as the antique and the Christian. It is a question, apparently, of multiplicity and detail. For if we compare the finished work of, say, Sophocles and Dante, it is impossible not to admit the overpowering superiority of Dante in respect of the manifold which he comprehends, and that æsthetically, within his artistic whole. We have had occasion, before, to compare the mind of Dante with the mind of Shakespeare ; and we were perhaps agreed that the former could not compare with the latter in breadth. The quality of Dante's mind, then, which we are trying to define, must be thought rather as intensive than as extensive. It is indeed qualities of intensiveness which characterise the mediæval mind as a whole, and which, appearing in their own way in mediæval art, impart their peculiar illumination.

The problem of multiplicity so far as it is met successfully by the mediæval consciousness becomes one of its values—perhaps the highest of its values. The achievement of mediæval Christianity was its assimilation of content. It saw that there were more issues in heaven or earth than the antique mind had dreamt of.

ART AND THE UNCONSCIOUS

A re-valuation or a trans-valuation of enormous import had been made through the insistence of the claim towards the individuality of *every* individual. It is obvious, however, that this recognition of the new claim created a problem of a totally new kind. It created a sense of responsibility that could almost be expressed in terms of the increased manifold of the social world that had, on the external side, to be organised. Moral and social organisation of this kind, however, must also be given in more individual terms than that of social structure or social relationships. It must also be expressed in terms of the character and development of the morally responsible individual himself. What, therefore, expresses itself on the outward side as a new problem of organisation, as an increase of extension of the field where moral relationship had to be exhibited, expresses itself on the side of the individual as a new problem of intensive values. Negatively, the types of conduct enjoined by the Christian conscience involved the denial of many forms of expression of man's nature that in a more pagan world would have been freely admitted. The entrammelling of speculative thought by dogmatic limitation is one example of this repression, and so far as it goes, an excellent one. The suggestion that part, at all events, of the value of mediæval thinking is to be credited to the severity of the limitations within which it had to move will raise the question of the positive aspect of what negatively appears as repression.

The limitation of the sensuous enjoyment of life which takes place through, or co-ordinate with, the advent of the Christian consciousness, is usually taken as the most typical aspect of the mediæval attitude. Too exclusive stress is often placed upon this aspect of mediæval Christianity ; it is nevertheless a very significant one, and for our purposes, important.

In so far as there is repression of any side of man's nature, there would appear all the phenomena, of whatever kind, that in general have been shown to be co-ordinate with repression—dreams, phantasies, fantastic thought systems, or what not. In so far as it is sensation and the immediately sensuous that is in abeyance, the phenomena of dreams, etc., will take on a specific character. It has been shown in the chapter on the Nature and Origin of the Imagination, that image, in a certain definite sense, represents the obverse of sensation. It is as though the psychic material or energy which would condition sensation or sustain it from within, being unable to find an expression through sensation or perception, or in Bergson's language, to insert itself within perceptions, develops specifically as images. The inhibition of sensation, that is to say, means an enrichment of the image content of the mind. Or otherwise, we may view the matter as if man's inherited psychical potentialities, his archetypes, in the sense of the archetype already defined, were capable of differentiation in two directions. They might, on the one hand, find expression in sensation and perception, or on the other hand, in the formation of images, or more generally, of the imagination. In so far as the first avenue of expression should be unavailable, they would go to reinforce the image content of the mind. In so far as much of this content might only find expression in dreams, or in any relatively archaic and undifferentiated form of experience, it would be quite correct to say that they furnish the content of the unconscious.

In so far, then, as such contrast can be drawn between the antique and the mediæval ; and in so far as it may be true to assert that the latter denotes an attitude of repression on the side of sensuous enjoyment, so far forth will there be a fuller content in the mediæval unconscious. The mediæval mind is thus in possession of a source of energy, of a potentiality, not possessed by the antique. This last proposition is one of extraordinary significance.

For there is a tendency among ourselves who review the history of the Christian movement to write down its main intention as a failure. Yet even Nietzsche avoided this error. For if he protested hatred of Christianity, he also perceived " the fine tension of the middle ages," which was begotten through the Christian attitude ;   and clearly if this attitude be a condition of intensive development, it is something whose values have to be recognised, were it only in the sphere of art. So far, therefore, from viewing the advent of Christianity upon Europe as a disaster, we must view it as *at least* something that engendered the very highest possibilities towards art—towards an art that in point of intensive qualities, at all events, should altogether eclipse the greatest art of the ancient world. Sophocles and Dante ! How different ! And yet the values that are Sophocles' could be realised only *before* the Christian era.

The apparent loss resulting from the denial of one side of life is really a gain, or at least the condition of further and new possibilities of life. We might almost say that there was a conflict between the immediate gratification of sense and the formation of a new *organon* of the spirit.

This conflict of the Christian ages between the immediacy of sensation and the discovery of other potentialities of mind naturally led to a profoundly different relation between the sexes from that which obtained in the antique world. This is the most important implication of all in the conflict between the values of immediacy, as, e.g., sensation, and the value of things not immediately present, but to be

attained or developed through a more or less protracted experience.

In so far as the orientation of man to woman was
necessarily less naïve and immediate in the Christian
world, we should find the same repression of one side
of his nature together with the genesis or at least the
development of that other side of it, the side remote
from that which is repressed. From one point of
view we must, of course, attach the higher value to
the more naïve, simple and direct relationship. But,
on the other hand, the problem and the stumbling-
block of the ancient world was the absence of spirituality in the relationship of man to woman. With
the advent of Christianity, the simplicity and directness of the relation were lost. Its qualities of fact,
of naïvete, of immediacy were lower. But on the
other hand the relationship was enriched by a new
content which at its highest, at all events, was certainly beyond the reach of the ancient world.

The mediæval world, does indeed show an amazing
enrichment of the spiritual side of man's nature in his
relationships. The greater mediæval artists show
this intensive development of spirituality in an
unmistakeable way. Dante may be surpassed by
Shakespeare or by Homer in range and breadth,
but he surpasses them both in the intensity of his
vision.

With Dante, literature has become our topic;
and it should not escape us that the relation of the
sexes and their orientation to each other is of unique
importance for literature among the arts. It is
always dangerous to assign a special function to a
particular art. Art is so full of surprises. Yet I
think we should state, and do careful justice to, the
proposition that what literature and, in special,
poetry, has always been striving after is the intuition
of human relationships. Architecture, clearly, cannot

do this at all ; nor can painting do it as well as literature, nor can music. The two latter arts may do it to some extent or in certain ways. Music, no doubt, can do it intensively, though otherwise under very narrow limitations. But none of these can, on any view, alike comprehend and fathom the soul of men and women in their relationship to each other as the art of literature can. From the first book of the *Iliad* to the last book of the *Forsyte Saga*, this is what literature has been trying to do all the time.

The great literary intuition of the relation of man to woman as developed through mediæval Christianity is the work of Dante—chiefly the *Vita Nuova* and the *Comedia*. In Dante s relation to Beatrice, there is an almost unfathomably rich content ; and this is what gives the poem its unique importance in respect of the relation of literature to the unconscious.

Going back, for a moment, to an earlier point of view, we saw that it was impossible to consider the Beatrice of the *Vita Nuova* or of the *Divina Comedia* as just the real Beatrice Portinari and nothing more. We had to think of her as a subjective figure in Dante himself—that part of Dante " that revealed him to himself." We found also that in another context we had to modify that general conclusion and that we had to regard the subjective figures of the poet's mind as not altogether independent of the men and women he had known. Bosanquet expresses this interpretation of the inner by the outer, or of the outer by the inner with a singular simplicity and clearness. " The selves," he says, " who figure in the poem have all rendered up their content to the great experience which was the poet's mind, and are constituent parts of it." He goes on to add, " None the less it is necessary for its effectiveness as a poem, that they should be regarded as acting and thinking beings." That they should be *regarded* as acting and thinking beings—is this enough ? For we have to remember how strong the purely historical consciousness was in Dante, and it is possible also that Beatrice Portinari did actually walk about the streets of Florence and was personally known to, and loved by, Dante. While, therefore, we might not need to say whether Beatrice is most to be taken as a figure of the inner life or as a person of the outer, we do need to keep in mind the twofold character of her being. She is *both* within and without.

But, after all, is it possible to refrain from asking whether she is most to be taken subjectively or as the real Beatrice ? For the Beatrice of the *Comedia* lives on in the experience of Dante long after the real Beatrice is dead. The writing of the *Comedia*, indeed, one feels inclined to think, was conditioned by her death. For us who review the whole process it is scarcely possible, I think, to evade the judgment that the Beatrice of the poem is far more subjective than objective ; while for Dante himself—and this is the essential matter—it is impossible to say whether she is subjective only or a real existence in her own right. For the most part, we feel, she is taken as real. But the doubtfulness—the absence of differentiation within the poet's own consciousness—is accurately exhibited in the words of *The Convito*—" Beatrice Beata who now lives in Heaven with the Angels, and on Earth in my Heart."[1]

Now it is just this attitude of Dante that can be taken as typical of the mediæval art consciousness, and all that is most significant in it. The Beatrice that is in the soul is confused with the real Beatrice, and so the subjective Beatrice is projected into heaven.

There is no other instance in literature where the whole structure of a poet's work is supposed to depend on the historical reality of the principal

[1] *Convito*, II., 2.

woman character. Compare Shakespeare : Miranda may, indeed, be for Shakespeare in the words of a modern critic, " a new function of consciousness." But there is no question either of confusing or identifying Miranda with a living lady whom Shakespeare knew. So with Goethe in whom both Margaret and Helena are perhaps more subjective than any corresponding figure in Shakespeare. There is again no confusion, no attempted identification of Margaret or Helena with women of the poet's acquaintance. In short, Beatrice has a supposed historical reality for Dante—a reality taken for granted in no other instance to the same extent.

Further than this, however. What applies to Beatrice applies to the whole poem. The entire structure of the *Comedia* depends upon the supposition of the historical reality of all its characters. A few minor exceptions like the heroes of Greek mythology scarcely call for specific reservation. In other words, Dante has acquired an intensity of historical consciousness that had never been reached before by the mediæval mind—if doubtfully reached anywhere by the antique. Dante is the source of the modern historical consciousness.

It is in terms of this consciousness that we can state the problem which gave rise to Dante's conflict, and which conditions his vision in the *Comedia*.

All religions have insisted upon their historic origin, or upon the historical reality of the hero or the celestial mother or the redeemer. But not in all religions has the conception of historical reality played the part which it has done in Christianity. Christianity has been the religion of the West. It stands in marked contrast to those of Egypt or of the further East. Now the West has, in distinction to the East, the strongest possible sense of historical fact. When the proposition is made by the Western mind that some thing or person is historically real, it means it with a vigour and force and clearness almost inapprehensible to the East. The typical Eastern mind would think it foolish—and very rightly so, from its own standpoint—to dispute about anything so insignificant as a fact of history. Not so, the West ; and if the West maintains that Christ was a real personage in history, it means a very great deal by that statement ; and all this it must have meant to Dante. The incarnation was the central fact of history ; but certainly to Dante it was a historical fact.

Added to this, or rather as part and parcel of it, there is his keen scientific interest. Nor must it be forgotten in estimating the æsthetic effect of his poem, that in such a canto as that about the spots on the moon, he really thought he was solving a scientific problem. The physical universe was something that, for Dante, had the same kind of reality as history. His universe is spatial and material, whatever it may be besides.

The unrealised, the content of the unconscious is alway projected. We have seen how rich and how relatively profound this unconscious had become for the mediæval. This unconscious manifold, therefore, is projected on to what is so well suited to bear that projection, viz., the spatial and material universe. Heaven and Hell and Purgatory are therefore *in this universe.* Or in other words, the whole problem of good and evil in Dante's own soul is worked out in terms of Earth and Heaven, in terms of concentric spheres revolving the one within the other.

But moral experience here and now is too real a thing quite to be banished to the ' other ' world, to be entirely projected into that other. The universe, therefore, falls apart into two—this world, and the other world ; present experience upon earth, and the future—of punishment, purification and redemption. The whole universe suffers this division ; but the moral universe shows it most clearly.

The classic exposition of this dualism in the poem has been given by Bosanquet[1]—an instance, among several, of that unsurpassable union of philosophical insight and sensibility with which he always speaks of Dante. For our purpose, however, it is important to see how the dualism affects Dante's rendering of the various *characters* in the poem. The dualism of the universe means, in psychological terms, division within the poet's own soul ; and this division finds expression in the ambiguous status of every character within it. It is never clear in what relation any given figure belongs to the soul of Dante himself, and in what relation, to the real world of history. This dubiety is especially intensified with regard to the figure of the woman, Beatrice, who appears in the poem in a fashion so unparallelled by any other work of literary art.

The significance of this fact will become clearer when we examine the method of artists of an equal rank with Dante, but of a later age.

[1] *History of Æsthetic*, Chap. VII.

CHAPTER III

THE MUSIC OF GERMANY AND THE LITERATURE OF ENGLAND

Love is my sin.
SHAKESPEARE

The hindrance lieth within himself.
MÊISTER ECKHARD

(1)

As art passes from the age of Dante and Giotto, it develops more and more power of representative technique. It becomes, in a very real sense, burdened with its own capabilities of delineating the objects of the outer world and with the variety of the world it has thus to portray

This is true especially of painting. It is a proposition that has not as yet any significance *apropos* of music. For that art is still in the making. What the modern world understands by music has scarcely come to birth before Palestrina. It is true our interest being so focussed on Italy, the musical achievements of the northern races of the time, especially of England and Flanders, are apt to slip out of mind. It is nevertheless perfectly easy to state an almost extreme form of the contrast between the older art of painting and the younger art of music at the time of the Renaissance. The contemporary artists, Michael Angelo and Palestrina, will serve better than any other representative minds to typify this contrast.

There is a strong tendency in present-day art criticism to judge Angelo with immoderate severity. This tendency is quite comprehensible, if my suggestion is right that the profounder artistic and critical instincts of our age go out to more ' primitive ' forms of art than that of the late Renaissance. Art like that of the Byzantine period, or of the Giottesque, is what it craves ; and with this craving, I have no quarrel—except, indeed, that I take the word, primitive, to be something of a misnomer. The fact, however, that Angelo and the later Florentines and Venetians have not the qualities of the ' primitives ' ; and that all the greatest of them have positively to stagger under this burden of representative technique, does not seem to me to put them outside the pale of art. They may stagger and groan, but they are giants and not dwarfs. Some of them are even colossi.

Michael Angelo's work, terrifically powerful as its effect is and will always be upon human sensibility, does lack the ' primitiveness' and purity of form of which some contemporary criticism is so exclusively in search. That it has other values—values, too, that keep it within the sphere of art—which remain after every formal criterion of this kind has been applied, I am quite sure.

But for our present purpose, it is enough to observe that the fulness of the intellectual and emotional resource which belongs alike to Angelo's genius and to the age in which he lived, constitutes a disentegrating force within those ' primitive ' forms of beauty in which art tends to rest ; and towards which, it may perhaps be admitted, it ought always to strive. It is possible, for example, to put into words a great deal of the religious and emotional content of the famous fresco on the roof of the Sistine Chapel. This has been done in a remarkable way by J. A. Symonds or by Romain Rolland.

Criticism tends to play round art of this kind ; for of course it offers a far easier problem to the critical function which is bound to make use of words. There

is here, too, a great danger. It is the danger of being
partial in the choice of art upon which scrutiny is to
be directed. The temptation is so obvious to single
out those types of art towards which it is an easy
matter to arouse the sensibility through language,
and to evade those other types whose formal character
precludes this facile method. In so far, however, as
criticism, by whatever fashion, achieves the goal of a
genuine æsthetic apprehension, it is justified. We
cannot, therefore, condemn either the art of Michael
Angelo or the criticism of Rolland because there
happens to be a certain facility of approach in
language. When, for example, Rolland summarises
his account of the fresco by saying that the prevailing
and final emotion of the whole gigantic work is *fear*,
he is simply saying something that is true, relevant
and vital. He has placed his finger upon the very
point of incidence of the religious forces upon the
artistic work. He just feels the bankruptcy of
Angelo's religious faith, and exhibits that very
bankruptcy as the source of his artistic power. Or,
with more psychological accuracy, we might say that
he seizes upon the central issue of Angelo's conflict and
shows how the conflict gives the motive power towards
that kind of art for which Angelo had the appropriate
genius. In the fresco there is an immensely large
content. It is so large that it bursts asunder the
beautiful, naïve, ' primitive ' forms of art. It is a
disintegrating force, this culture of Angelo's, but it
does not disintegrate to the extent of forcing the
resultant product quite outside the domain of art.
The fresco is, in some sense, one of the most beautiful
things in the world. But Angelo's was the last
artistic mind in Europe that could stand the obtrusion
of this vast culture-content into art. After him, it
bursts asunder all the limits that render possible that
type of painting.

ART AND THE UNCONSCIOUS

How definitely certain judgments can be made about Angelo! For example, there is, in him, and in particular in this fresco of the Sistine Chapel, a magnificent acceptance and worship of tradition—of the very idea of the church. No doubt, too, there was in him a profound inner scorn of the Church, of its Popes and its Authority. But making due allowance, there is a delight in all that hierarchy of prophets and saints, an eagerness in making Vergil the prophetic minister of Christ, a worship of the power of tradition, in short, from which he could not have dreamed of freeing himself.

The church and its authority are far better expressed and enforced, as far as art is concerned, through the visible·—and tangible—than in any other way. The idea of incarnation is made concrete in paint or stone. Architecture and the arts generally in which Angelo excelled are therefore integrally bound up with the ideas of authority and of incarnation in a very concrete sense. The misunderstanding of Angelo would be a profound one that supposed him to have freed himself from that, even taking into account all the paganism of St. Peter's and all the scepticism of his culture.

How difficult by contrast it is to make judgments of this kind about Palestrina and his music! The art of Palestrina is all that that of Angelo is not. Angelo is struggling with a multiplicity of content that is far too great for even his colossal strength. Palestrina, whatever be his artistic problem, has no difficulty of this kind. In the Marcellus Mass he has simply to take the old words and set them to his own new music. And the result is so incredibly simple! so incredibly 'primitive,' if there is anything enlightening in that word.

The reason is that Palestrina's religion stands to his music in so entirely different a relation from that in which Angelo's conflict stands to his fresco. In

the genius of Palestrina, enlisted as it was by Pope
Marcellus directly for the service of the church, there
is something that spontaneously and immediately
elucidates the spirituality of the age about to be
initiated. On one side Palestrina is more Christian
and belongs to an older religious generation than
Angelo ; on another side he is more in the future and
vests more of himself in the coming age.

The incidence of the religious forces of the age on
the new art—music—is quite different from their
incidence on the elder arts. For the purposes of
music, the idea of incarnation, for example, has
become more generalised, more spiritualised, in a
sense, even more rationalised. As the theologians
used to say, the accent has been transferred from
incarnation to atonement ; and this change of accent
gives the key to the artistic mode in which the religious
ideas and the religious emotions are to express themselves.

In the beautiful passage, for example, in the *Missa
Papæ Marcelli* accompanying the words, "Qui propter
homines . . . et homo factus est — " the traditional
idea of the incarnation is, of course, present ; but
because we are dealing with music and not painting
any concrete representation of the Christ is *ipso facto*
impossible. The voices may tell you about Christ,
but they cannot present any form of his body to the
senses, and so far forth the impression of concrete
reality of incarnation is diminished. This principle
runs through the entire contrast of music with painting
and sculpture.

This explains why it was that at the Renaissance,
the time of these arts as the great force they had been
in the world came to an end. It was impossible for
the age to accept the conception of incarnation in the
way in which it had been accepted for the thousand
years preceding. And generalising beyond the theo-

logical concept of incarnation, the age had begun to recognise its projection of the 'other' world; or had begun to make the discovery of the division within the unity of the mind and to search for a means towards " the restitution of this divided unity."

The simplest formulation of this transition is, I think, given in the strange rapidity with which the glory of the stained glass dies out in the Gothic cathedral and the sudden diminishing of its spirituality in the fourteenth and fifteenth centuries. It is as if the Gothic spirit of transcendence had failed to effect anything further along the lines of representation of a visible Christ or a visible Madonna. And, of course, all the critics whose scope has been restricted to the arts of architecture, sculpture, painting and glass work have spoken of the decadence of art during these centuries—from the fourteenth to the sixteenth. But art is not really decadent. Almost before the magnificence of colour had begun to die out of the windows, John of Dunstable had discovered the new art of counterpoint—early in the fourteenth century. This new art contained the whole power of the future. The essentials of the art spirit are withdrawn from the windows to the music. That is all.

It is not unfair, however to represent the greatest period of European music as initiated about 1600. The Teutonic movement in music from then onwards is the only movement in art that can be placed in rivalry with the literature of the English Renaissance. It staggers the imagination that German music and English dramatic literature should have burst forth about the same time, and apparently out of the same aboriginal Teutonic stem.

GERMANY AND ENGLAND

(2)

Turning to Bach, I should first of all attempt to relate his pre-eminence in music to the subjective character of the art. It is in pure music, at its most typical, that there is least of all a sense of outer objects. Experience, here, is least of all an experience of objects ; and here, most of all, can meaning be attributed to the idea of experience as such and not as of something.

The music of Bach was founded upon the chorale. It can be regarded almost as a development of that. The old German chorale which, as Nietzsche said, came out of the abyss of the Reformation is significant in the history of religion as a means of expressing the directness of the relation between the soul and God. It can be contrasted, here, with the forms of worship of the Latin church. Through the chorale, the Christian confession of sin has changed in character. The German chorale is perhaps more typically burdened by a sense of personal guilt than any other form of worship hitherto. In Bach this sense of sin with its corresponding direct claim upon God is carried to an extent, I think, unknown in music either before or after him. When he was 17 years old, he wrote the chorale-prelude, " Have mercy upon me, O Lord," which is so extraordinary for a boy of that age. It is as though it were a literal translation into music of one of the Pauline epistles. And here I should do my argument the justice of noting that this was my own mental comment when first I discovered it without knowing what the hymn was to which it was the organ prelude.

The climax in the musical treatment of this theme—the sense of sin—may be typified, for example, in the great double chorus in chorale form, " O man, thy grievous sin bemoan " in the Matthew passion music.

This chorale has indeed received many renderings by Bach. It is possible that it gripped him more completely than any other. However that may be, I mention the setting in the Matthew passion music because there is a certain point in contrasting it with the music of the *Kyrie Eleison* in the B minor mass. For the latter expresses more the generalised tragic emotion of all suppliants from every kindred and nation and tongue ; whereas this chorus based upon the chorale, " O Mensch, bewein dein Sünde gross," has that strange, unparalleled quality of expressing the personal Christian consciousness, its personal grief and its personal exaltation. Now the music with which we are dealing is the only ecclesiastical music that can stand in rivalry with Latin church music. Bach, indeed, borrows the forms of the Latin church and his greatest success of all is in the Mass. It is quite true that the Mass in B minor is specifically different from Latin music either of the Italian or of the Germans themselves. But even in Bach there is a contrast between the more generalised emotion of the *Kyrie Eleison* in the B minor Mass and the more personal outpouring of the individual—or local— experience in the St. Matthew chorus.

In these cases, we have a cue afforded us by the difference between the Latin and the German form of worship and between the Latin and the German words. But I think we can take up this cue and follow the same line of differentiation in Bach's purely instrumental music. I think, for example, that the same contrast will be found to some extent between the organ works that follow the spirit of the St. Anne fugue and those that follow the spirit of the great B minor.

At all events, I should certainly venture to connect artistic emotion with the historical religious consciousness of the time, in the instance of the St. Anne fugue.

It begins with a passage in five part polyphony that in every way resembles the chorale, in spirit and form. In reminiscence and emotion it takes us back to nothing save the chorale. It is, therefore, impossible to dissociate the last third of the figure—surely the most unalloyed expression of joy in the whole range of music—from just that religious emotion and just those religious memories. It is at all events a religious joy, as exuberant as religious. We have scarcely a logical ground for taking the further step and saying that it is the expression of the sense of liberation and spiritual freedom that belongs to those times at their best. But we may feel, perhaps, that the truth lies in that general direction.

The same thing may be illustrated from his treatment of the *Magnificat*. The Leipzig *Magnificat*, for example, forcibly exhibits the contrast between the way in which the idea of the Virgin appears in the religious consciousness after the Reformation and the way in which the Catholic worshipper conceived her. From the very conditions of the art of painting, she is, of course, presented in the most personal form. But over and above the more impersonal sensibility towards the image of the Virgin which would be bound to accrue from a musical as opposed to a visible symbol, the depersonalisation of the Virgin is— in this *Magnificat*--at its height. Especially, so it seems to me, in the *Et Exultavit*, the emotion that is properly to be ascribed to a woman has become a function of the worshipper in general. Psychologically, the image of the Virgin is apprehended in its true nature, *i.e.*, as subjective, as in the soul ; and consequently it is not projected into anything external, and so far forth there is secured a more complete understanding of the soul by itself. It is the difference between the age of Dante and the age of Bach.

Artists so different as Bach and Dante are thus

directly related along the line of a perfectly articulate evolution. In Dante, it is not known whether the image of the woman is subjective or not, and in so far as he is confused, the image is necessarily projected on to that supposed to be without. In Bach, there is no confusion, or at least there is a far higher degree of recognition of the essential subjectivity of the image. There is therefore a higher degree of self-relation or of self-unity.

It is thus impossible to evade the question how the inwardness of Bach's music is to be correlated to its motivation. In so far as we summarise this motivation as the problem of sin and redemption—the problem of the *Erlösung* that has always loomed so large in the German mind—we may very easily exhibit it as having issued here in the most inward expression that European art has given it.

(3)

If we turn to the Elizabethans, to Shakespeare and Milton, to Webster and Sidney, the *saltus* that we have to make seems for a moment too vertiginous. The contrast between the temperaments of the epochs or between the forms of expression they choose, is almost too startling. Certainly, the English look outward ; their orientation, if ever it could be said of any race in their characteristic art, is towards men and women and nature—to the outer object, always, but above all to the human object. Yet they also, in their own way, encountered the problem of sin ; and their expression in this regard is as poignant as Bach's. Only, it is so very different. For with them it appears with respect to outer objects and human relationships. For the German, the problem of *Erlösung* does not arise so much in the orientation of man to his outer world or

to his fellow human beings as through the inner relations of mind and heart. Or rather, wherever it be
that it arises, it is *recognised* in that inner relation.
For the Elizabethans the sense of sin was the sense of
ineffective outer relationship.

Of course, this is a formulation of a tendency, the
summary of a racial type. It will be easy enough to
discover instances that point in the contrary direction.
But such instances, however clear in themselves, must
not be allowed to obscure the prevailing tendencies of
each country—which do indeed prevail so effectually
and so forcefully.

The negative instances, however, and the inter-
mediate cases are, after all, too important to ignore,
and too significant. Where, for example, shall we
place the music of Bach's contemporary, Handel ?
This, so English in character, springing to birth, even,
on English soil, and so acceptable to the English
temperament, might indeed serve as a kind of mediating term between the two types of art. Samuel
Butler links together his two beloved divinities,
Shakespeare and Handel, by pointing out that it was
an English bishop, who, quoting Shakespeare, said of
Handel : " This man doth fear God, howsoever it
seems not in him by some large jests he will make."

And what of Purcell ? Or of Byrd ? And what of
the English madrigal ? The latter is no doubt the
counterpart of the German chorale and the forms of
music that grew out of it. For when the English
become sad, they sing madrigals ; and when the
Germans become gay, they sing cantatas. There
would still be a very long way to go before they meet ;
and who could catch the spirit of English music ? Of
the two essences, the English is undoubtedly the
subtler and the more ethereal, and the more impossible
to call by any name.

Yet it is not impossible to grasp, and to hold, the

proposition that what makes the utterance of the Elizabethans so poignant is this reflection upon the failure of the earthly and tangible relationships. The beautiful line of Sidney's sonnet might be taken as emblematic :—

Leave me, O Love, that reachest but to dust.

The whole literature of the sonnet is, indeed, of peculiar significance in this epoch. And we are not to discard even what seems childish and artificial in it. It should be taken rather as a prelude to that larger utterance about human love, and human destiny—individual love and individual destiny—that single it out from every other period of European literature through the peculiar richness of its feeling for those individual things. The sonnet is the precocious expression of the youthfulness of an age in which for its maturity individual relationships were to take on new forms and present new problems. But the enormously rich content given by Shakespeare to this aspect of relationship makes most claim upon our attention. The sonnet sequence must indeed be viewed as the preface to his dramatic work. It is the record of that phase of his experience in which the bewilderment and sorrow over the failure of relationship is still personal and before it has passed into the more universal form of emotion that is the mainspring of the greatest of his dramatic work. This sonnet sequence I should incline to call the most remarkable personal document in literature.

It is enough, here, to note the quick following up of those passionate assertions towards the end of the sequence about the permanence of love by the confession of bankruptcy and disillusion :—

Love is not love
Which alters when it alteration finds,
Or bends with the remover to remove—

and then the last sonnet, in which the author seeks to

carry off his own defeat—the mockery with which he salutes the illusion of his having

> . . . laid great bases for eternity
> Which proves more short their waste or ruining.

With the theme of the sonnets in our mind, then, we turn to the dramatic movement which was the main contribution of England to Renaissance art.

Perhaps nowhere in the whole history of art does the admitted fact of the licentiousness of the artist, together with the power of his art, so thrust itself forward upon the thinking mind or so relentlessly clamour for explanation as it does in the Elizabethan drama. There had been a sinister tradition of evil at times among the artists of the later Renaissance in Italy. But that period we incline to call decadent perhaps on that very account. In any case, we have no sense of the exuberant vitality of a new movement that we find in the England of Elizabeth. If anything can be said of the dramatic movement of the sixteenth century, it is that it was bursting with sheer vitality. Then men were alive, and so was art. The problem of evil in relation to art is therefore presented in this epoch with a peculiar simplicity and reality.

It was the genius of England to have power over the outer object; the highest phase of this power is represented in the development of human relations. And it is just this power over the outer object that lies behind English literature, and through which we must look for the inspiration of English poetry. With all its magnitude and majesty, Elizabethan and Jacobean literature never quite reaches the depth of Athenian tragedy or of the *Divina Comedia*. I do not see how this claim can be made for it, just because Shakespeare excels the author of the *Agamemnon* or *The Comedia* in so many ways other than in depth.

If we exclude Goethe and Keats—or again, in

another kind, Dostoevsky—it is easy to secure for
Dante the place of the profoundest of European poets.
The beauty of his work comes through its depth. It
might be possible—perhaps easy—to claim for
Aeschylus that he outreaches any of the Elizabethans
in depth. But for all that, Shakespeare and Milton
remain unchallenged in beauty—Milton in passages,
Shakespeare in passages, and also in certain plays as a
whole. Now, if this eminence is not attained through
depth of insight—and I cannot help feeling that it is
wrong to try to substantiate it that way—how has it
been attained ? I think the true answer is that it has
come through the reflection, in poetry, of the English
power of handling the outer object—its genius for
immediate, vital rapport with all sorts and conditions
of men and women. That is indeed the genius of
England ; and it will have its own form and its own
reflection among her artists—especially among her
poets. Her political genius—how admirably, how
absurdly, it is reflected in Milton—yet with what
magnificent literary effect !

In Milton, indeed, this peculiar reflection of the
English temperament, is fraught with a kind of
anomaly. The invocation, for example, at the opening
of the third book of *Paradise Lost* is surely unequalled
for pure beauty in the literature of any language.
Yet students of poetry, from generation to generation,
have gone to Milton looking for depth of spiritual
insight. And they have always had to come away
empty and disappointed. For in this passage of
resplendent beauty sustained through nearly sixty
lines, perhaps a longer flight of undiminished inspiration
than can be found elsewhere in European poetry—in
this unsurpassed perfection of the English language
there is certainly nothing that can be called depth.
Why, then is it so beautiful ? The answer, it seems to
me, must be that though depth of insight is one of the

things that can, if the conditions are otherwise favourable, give beauty in poetry ; there are other factors, too, through which beauty will come.

My supposition is, then, that the gifts of the race to which Milton belonged, and that I express briefly as its power over the outer object, is inherited by him, poet and studious scholar though he was, as only a student could inherit it. But this curious inheritance of the student-poet has given us poetry of an unique and unparalleled kind. I should suppose that the beauty of the passage in question arises out of those racial qualities in him which enabled him to live passionately in the objects of his love without caring whether or not it was possible to bring the different passions into harmony within the compass of a single soul. In his art he views the different incompatible objects—the Antique, the Hebrew, the English political conflict— as it were through different facets of his mind, and there is no singleness of vision. It is a purely kaleidoscopic vision—crystalline, jewelled, ununified. There is, no doubt, in each isolated case, a perfect blending of the unconscious with the objective vision ; but " those thoughts that wander through eternity " never come to rest long enough upon any one object to let the floods of the unconscious pour themselves out upon it.

> In my flight
> Through utter and through middle darkness borne
> With other notes than to th' Orphean Lyre '
> I sung . . . . . .

If only Milton could have gazed or listened steadily enough, if only he could have given himself time, to hear that Lyre in relation with those *other* notes, to comprehend their resonance within a single harmony ! But this implies a self-knowledge and a self-intuition that he never could have had, and for which, after all, it were vain to wish.

ART AND THE UNCONSCIOUS

With all its breadth and variety, there is one thing in Elizabethan and Jacobean literature that I think we must admit to be of pre-eminent importance; and that is *the death of the Hero*. For, after all, it is dramatic tragedy that we must take as central and typical in the kind of Art which now comes up for our consideration. Here I find myself committed to what looks like a contradiction; but since I must at this point bring together two sides of the matter that appear at first sight incompatible, I pause to explain as clearly as may be what these aspects are.

I have suggested that the art of Milton and Shakespeare was the art of a race that showed great command over external things—over armies and navies, for example, and political organisations. And yet I have committed myself to the belief that the spirit of tragedy is the most inward of the poetic gifts. How, then, does this theme, the death of the Hero which I have taken to be pre-eminent for the epoch, stand between the outwardness of the racial spirit and the inwardness of the tragic spirit?

For ancient tragedy, it was sufficient if, in the language of Aristotle, the hero was one " who is highly renowned and prosperous—a personage like Oedipus, Thyestes, or other illustrious men of such families." Doing, perhaps, a little more justice to the hero of ancient tragedy, we might say, he had, in some way to be a great man—to have some great qualities of character. But that is enough. Oedipus is indeed quite fairly typical. The difference then between Greece and England in this respect is that the latter must exhibit her hero as great in the attitude of command—command over men and things—and over their complexity and the multiplicity of their detail.

In Bosanquet's *Logic* there will be found the characteristic remark that even the Greek intellect in its prime, or Greek art at its best, has not the many-sided concreteness that belongs to Shakespeare or Goethe, Raphael or Turner. Now I suggest that nowhere is this many-sidedness so well exhibited by contrast as in the great soldier heroes of Shakespeare—Julius Cæsar, Othello, Coriolanus, Macbeth. And in the most subtle study of all—Hamlet—the hero is exhibited as possessing an extraordinary wealth of resource in his handling of things and his dealings with men. This is just what the English genius could do, this was just the artistic task it had to undertake. And if, in sheer profundity, it came short of Dante and Goethe and, I had almost said, of Keats, it certainly excelled all these in breadth and variety. The greater the breadth the fuller the concreteness and richness of detail in the setting forth of the heroic powers of command, the greater, one might naturally conclude, would be the difficulty of securing the inwardness which is the essence of the tragic spirit. But this inwardness is secured ; and to this extent that after all, Hamlet, as the tragic hero, is surpassed in depth in European literature by Faust alone.

But returning to the standpoint from which we viewed art as the interpretation of the outer by the inner and of the inner by the outer, we should have to say that the hero, Macbeth or Hamlet or Othello is part of Shakespeare himself. That would be true in any case ; and we must affirm and re-affirm that there was Macbeth in Shakespeare, and Hamlet and Othello and the other glorious and unfulfilled possibilities and failures. But when it is asserted that these heroes were part of Shakespeare himself it is not possible to say this quite in the same way or to think it on the same plane as when it was suggested that Beatrice was part of Dante himself. There may be many reasons why the two cases are not quite similar. One of them only we need here discuss.

The *Comedia* is a poem to be read in the seclusion of one's own room or to be enjoyed at most by two or three persons—perhaps most enjoyed by not more than two. Elizabethan tragedies are never really apprehended in their completeness apart from the stage and the enthusiasm of crowds of people experiencing together a common emotion. But not every good play meets with the approval of the audience on its own merits. Apart from other reasons, the difficulty of presentation of a play of a former epoch is considerable, and as a rule prevents to some extent the perfect rapport of players and audience. On the other hand the attitude of the contemporary audience is a vital condition of the finest dramatic art. And the strong appetite of the Elizabethan crowd for the Elizabethan play fulfils this condition in a way that it perhaps has been rarely fulfilled elsewhere or at other times.

The idea of the naval or military or political hero would carry with it a powerful emotion in those times. We have therefore to say that in the spectators no less than in the Marlowes or Shakespeares the sense of the hero is potent ; and that Macbeth or Tamberlaine are, psychologically, in those very spectators themselves.

It is, I think, necessary to emphasise the enthusiasm of the age for the dramatic and the spectacular, for the court and the pageant. Rupert Brooke, in a delightful little sentence in his book on Webster, has spoken of the " arts of the theatre, creeping slowly out when religion has slept, as in the eighteenth century, or someti nes liberated by such splendid bursts of irreligion as pr duced the Elizabethan drama in England." What he calls " irreligion," I should certainly not so designate. The motive force behind was perhaps not Christian, but it does not follow that it was irreligious. At all events, there can be no question about the value of these "splendid bursts of irreligion." There is a quality in them not altogether different from the spirit of the martyrs, though the resultant action seem so different. Some things, history assures us, are worth dying for ; and we might, I think, accept the more easily her assurance that some things are worth living for. Waiving then for the present, the question whether we are to describe the Elizabethan genius for pageantry as religious or irreligious, the popular enthusiasm which lies behind a great epoch of dramatic art is something apart from which we cannot correctly state our problem of art.

No small part of the significance of this popular enthusiasm and of the intensely vital urge of the age towards the theatre is the daily awakening sense that the hero is in the soul itself ; and that through all the adventures of the soul it looks for the hero for its salvation ; but finally that the hero always fails it. The hero must always fail it. That is the essential of tragedy. But why is this ? Why must the hero always be defeated ?

There is nothing in æsthetic theory that has been so effectively handled as theory of tragedy. It is indeed the only part of that science that is not in its infancy. This fact is not to be regarded as something merely fortuitous in the development of European thought. We should rather seek to view it along the line of the argument which I have ventured to develop in preceding pages. Criticism and æsthetic encounter, as we have seen, their supreme difficulties in music. In literature with its critical tradition in Europe, dating at least from Aristotle's discussion of Athenian dramatic poetry, their task is far simpler and they are furnished with the results of centuries of investigation and reflection. I should say that the incidence of thought upon art is at its keenest and most effective when philosophical reflection is directed upon the tragic spirit. The literature of philosophy of our own age—say from the Romantic revival—is peculiarly rich in speculation on the nature of tragedy. I think it is Hegel here, who has gone furthest, and who merits most consideration. A. C. Bradley makes the remark that Hegel's *Theory of Tragedy* is the only work that the modern world has to set against Aristotle's poetics ; and Bradley has done for Hegel the vital service of freeing his work from the mere encumbrances of its dialectical form and of exhibiting its essential content with a reality and convincingness that Hegel's slavery to the artificial form of his dialectic tends to obscure. Bradley's treatment of Shakespearian tragedy is, therefore,. of peculiar value, combining as it does the depth of reflection that comes from a genuine philosophical heritage with the concrete actuality of English criticism.

With Bradley then I return once again to the sense of the moral order as the prime condition of tragedy. In contrasting tragedy with comedy—or with any other form of dramatic art—he makes what seems to me an essential point, viz., that the tragic spirit is not really reached unless the hero has that very defect of character that involves the catastrophe. In a non-tragic form of drama there can be found the more completely developed actor who escapes the mortal defect. But in tragedy this is not possible. With this I am in entire agreement. But it seems to me necessary to take this further step and to show that the hero must have this defect *in virtue of his greatness*. Defect of character that involves catastrophe does not constitute tragedy. The drama which is also tragic must exhibit the defect as *in virtue of* the very power or excellence or greatness of spirit that belongs to the hero.

Now this is the subjective appeal. The fundamental, eternal appeal which the tragic drama makes to the soul of man is in its power to show him that the tragedy of the soul happens no otherwise than through the soul's own excellence and gifts and genius.

But then the tragic drama is pleasure ; it is beautiful, and it was once at least, in a very specific and definite way religious. I do not think, indeed, the Elizabethan drama ought to be called religious in the sense in which Athenian drama was religious. Perhaps in the largest and ultimate sense we shall be able to call it religious. It was indeed

- the prophetic soul
Of the wide world dreaming on things to come.

But we could not interpret it as religious in any more specific sense. Yet in so far as it confronts the human soul with the secret of its own destiny ; and in so far as the soul is not repelled or set in any kind of antagonism, but becomes submissive and is uplifted, just in so far we do discover the essentials of the religious spirit—something that claims to be related more deeply and more completely to other manifestations of the same spirit. This claim is certainly not to be evaded.

Nor can it be said that the Elizabethan drama is religious in the sense in which the music of Bach is religious. For I think the student of music is in duty bound to contend that the form which the Christian religion happened to take in the seventeenth century did in a very direct and manifest way, inspire his choral works and his organ fugues. It would, of course be quite untrue, or rather absurd, to say that any form of religion which can be named, inspired the tragedies of Webster or of Shakespeare. That much we must state clearly in order that we may also be sure of such religious force as does really lie behind the apparently secular drama.

But when all is said, and when all allowances have been made, I should still wish to urge that there is a vital significance in the comparison we have tried to

draw between the two periods of culture as art-epochs.
For both, religious and moral authority in the old sense
had been swept away. For both, challenge is
made to the soul to find its own principle of
initiative and to voyage out alone into new and strange
seas of thought and emotion. But in reformation
music the demand is felt mainly for the soul to find its
relationship with itself. No doubt the problem of sin
and redemption is just that, in the last resort, all the
world over ; but in England there is the mediate
problem, so poignantly stated there, of the soul's
relationship with other souls. Hence the divergence
of the artistic spirit as it goes to find its expression in
Germany or England.

(5)

So we return once more to the divergent tendency
inherent in all art between its intuition as a symbol
that is to lead to the future and to a better life, and
its intuition as the discovery or creation of some
' eternal ' value—

> Out of the wash of days and temporal tide.

Art always presents this two-fold aspect.

Dr. Ernest Jones in his remarkable analysis of
Hamlet shows that the hero's conflict takes place
through his unrecognised identification with the
incestuous uncle. Through this identification, Hamlet
is himself guilty of incest in the sense in which Oedipus
is guilty, and yet it is he himself who is bound by a
moral necessity to punish the incestuous guilt by
death. Hence the incapacity for action with which
he is paralysed—an incapacity otherwise so out of
harmony with his character. Subject only to a
possible reservation about his use of the term, incest,

Dr. Jones' analysis is clear and convincing, so far as it goes, beyond any possibility of question. There is also an explicit recognition, as a preface to the analysis, of the æsthetic value of art apart from, or over and above, its interest as reflecting light upon the character of the artist.

Having gone so far, then, why should Dr. Jones altogether ignore the end of the play, that part of the action which begins with the mortal wounding of Hamlet ? For with the inevitableness of the death of the hero, the tragic issue changes. The charge is laid upon Horatio by the dying Hamlet to make clear the situation and to restore order within the state. At the same time, and together with this partial illumination, it is shown in the play that the illumination is, in its very nature, incomplete. It is clear, æsthetically, that the new knowledge, together with the limitation of that knowledge, belongs integrally to the play. They must be viewed within the whole æsthetic impression. They are essential to its beauty. Why does Horatio live, and make known ? Why must Hamlet die and the rest be silence ? The point at issue, it seems to me, is that the excellence of the hero is so integrally bound up with his defect, that there is no possibility of separation of excellence and defect *within the hero himself.* He dies ; and his problem of immortality remains unresolved. This means that the Hamlet in Shakespeare dies, and " the rest is silence."

If, then, the play of Hamlet be essentially an interpretation of Shakespeare's own experience through objects—through the world of men and women upon which he looked out, is it not essential that we should complete this interpretation of his mind by bringing back again within that mind whatever is meant by the enlightenment of Horatio and the silence of Hamlet. It is Hamlet who dies, not Shakespeare. But Horatio is the essential factor of enlightenment. Hence

Shakespeare lives and *can* live because he knows—
through Horatio. On the other hand, he knows
imperfectly. " The rest is silence."

It is not unlikely that for us who live three hundred
years after Shakespeare wrote, the knowledge of
Horatio will have another, and a greater, significance
than it had for Shakespeare. Nevertheless its import
is not, and can never be, so great as to amount to the
discovery of the unrevealed secret. It is as though the
boundaries between the knowledge of Horatio and the
unrevealed might shift, but not break down. The
knowledge, shall we say, will increase ; and this
domain of knowledge it is the function of critical
analysis to widen, and more thoroughly to explore. It
is the domain of ' the idea of conscious reflection '
within which many minds can enter. In virtue of this
entry into it, they may follow the artist and have their
vision in common with him. In so far, also, as the
domain has been widened and explored, they may have
a better approach to the object of his vision than even
he had himself. They may see further and more
deeply. The art consciousness of our own day may be
profound with respect to the art of the past. Though
we know Hamlet's secret in terms of an intimacy to
which Horatio could never have attained, Hamlet is
none the less admirable, nor the tragedy of Hamlet
less noble. The width or depth of the knowledge will,
of course, make a difference to the vision. If the play
is such that the widening and deepening knowledge
affords no change or novelty in the vision, conceivably,
with increasing knowledge, the play will pall. If on
the other hand—which is more likely—the deepening
and the widening of the ideational approach reveals
new things within the vision, the play will maintain its
old power, or command a new interest. Possibly it
may be the test of the greatest art that it maintains,
or deepens, its æsthetic appeal in proportion to the

richness of the consciousness in virtue of which approach to it is made.

I conceive it possible that the beauty of the *Sanctus* in Bach's mass is more intense for the deeper apprehension of the non-Christian consciousness than for the Christian.

Be that as it may, art must always move as between the enlightenment of Horatio and the silence of Hamlet. As thus moving between that knowledge and this silence, it may be exceedingly hard to tell whether it is most loved because of its illumination or because of what can never enter into the domain of knowledge. Its silence is, perhaps, after all, the supreme factor in its beauty. There is something that will never be disclosed.

> Thou still unravish'd bride of quietness !
> Thou foster-child of Silence . . .
> Thou, silent form ! dost tease us out of thought
> As doth eternity . . .

Of course, the silence is given in terms of harmony, a harmony so profound, and of instincts in the soul that move at so profound a depth, that we shall never be able to bring them to the light, or to say what they are. But since they are always there, and since their resonance may, at any time, be effected through the presence of the beauty of art, you may, if you like, call that beauty ' eternal.'

BIBLIOGRAPHY AND INDEX

*References only to proper names, and individual works of literature,
philosophy, art, architecture or music.*

BIBLIOGRAPHY AND INDEX

BIBLIOGRAPHY AND INDEX

240

BIBLIOGRAPHY AND INDEX